Joseph Nowinski, Ph.D., was born in Brooklyn, New York, in 1946. A graduate of Hofstra University, he did graduate work in clinical psychology at Syracuse University and the University of Connecticut, and post-doctoral training in sex therapy and research at the State University of New York at Stony Brook. He is currently Director of the Counseling Unit of the Human Sexuality Program, University of California San Francisco. In addition to teaching, training, and research, he maintains a private practice.

JOSEPH NOWINSKI

BECOMING SATISFIED

A MAN'S GUIDE TO SEXUAL FULFILLMENT

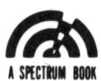
A SPECTRUM BOOK

PRENTICE-HALL, INC., Englewood Cliffs, N.J. 07632

Library of Congress Cataloging in Publication Data

NOWINSKI, JOSEPH.
   Becoming satisfied.

   (A Spectrum Book)
   Includes index.
   1.–Sex instruction for men. 2.–Sexual intercourse.
I.–Title.
HQ36.N68   613.9'6'024041   80-329
ISBN 0-13-073031-9
ISBN 0-13-073007-6 pbk.

Editorial/production supervision and interior design by Donald Chanfrau
Manufacturing buyer: Cathie Lenard

© 1980 by Prentice-Hall, Inc., Englewood Cliffs, New Jersey 07632

A SPECTRUM BOOK

All rights reserved.
No part of this book may be reproduced in any form
or by any means without permission in writing from the publisher.

10 9 8 7 6 5 4 3 2 1

Printed in the United States of America

PRENTICE-HALL INTERNATIONAL, INC., *London*
PRENTICE-HALL OF AUSTRALIA PTY. LIMITED, *Sydney*
PRENTICE-HALL OF CANADA, LTD., *Toronto*
PRENTICE-HALL OF INDIA PRIVATE LIMITED, *New Delhi*
PRENTICE-HALL OF JAPAN, INC., *Tokyo*
PRENTICE-HALL OF SOUTHEAST ASIA PTE. LTD., *Singapore*
WHITEHALL BOOKS LIMITED, *Wellington, New Zealand*

contents

preface ix

1
reassessing male and female sexuality 1

The Male Sexual Script 2   The Female Sexual Script 4
Scripts and Sexual Dysfunctions 6   Being Functional Versus Being
Fulfilled 17   Sexual Myths: Ideals Not to Live By 26
Summary 34

2
self-discovery 37
Sexual Scripts Versus Sexual Schemas 39 Dimensions of Sexual Interest 43 Male Sensuality 70 Summary 75

3
enhancing your sexual relationship 77
Sexual Communication 78 Expanding Sexual Repertoires 92 The Sexual Situation 100 Summary 105

4
developing your sexuality further 107
Letting Yourself Be Sexual 100 Appearances 113
Enjoying Yourself 118 Fantasy 122 Facilitating Sexual Expression 129 Sexual Histories 133 Summary 138

5
learning to relax 139
Tension and Relaxation 142 The Relaxation Technique 145 Building Body Awareness 151 Using the Relaxation Technique 155
Summary 157

6
overcoming sexual tension 158

Setting the Stage for Relaxation 159   Planning for Relaxation 167
Sensual Massage 168   Patterns of Intimacy and Sexual Fulfillment 174
Summary 188

7
overcoming fears of women 190

Sexual Shyness 191   Sexual Phobias 204   Summary 231

8
understanding erection problems 233

Assessing the Problem 235   Expecting the Possible: Sexual Desire and Erection Problems 240   Complications 243   Stumbling Blocks to Success 263   Summary 267

9
dealing with erection problems 269

Plan of the Program 270   Sexual Arousal and Erections 273

Understanding Desensitization 276
Desensitization Procedure for Erection Problems 278
Backsliding and What to Do About It 290
A Note for Single Men 297   Summary 304

10
learning to delay orgasm 306

Controlling Your Arousal: What to Expect 309   Channels of Stimulation and Sexual Arousal 310   Plan of the Program 314   Learning to Delay Orgasm 316
Summary 334

11
learning to accelerate orgasm 336

Setting Goals 337   Plan of the Program 337
Summary 344

index 345

preface

The goal of this book is to provide tools and guidelines that men can use to help improve the quality of their relationships, especially their sexual lives. It is based on the notion that what men want, sexually and otherwise, is more than what they have traditionally been offered. First, there are programs that can be used to overcome specific sexual difficulties and achieve specific goals, like keeping an erection, lasting longer, and reaching orgasm sooner. There are also programs and exercises, however, designed for broader objectives: to become more sensual; to learn to relax; to build intimacy and communication within relationships; and more. These are included in the belief that many men want not only to be sexually *functional*, but sexually *fulfilled* as well.

Feeling sexually fulfilled is not the same as being sexually functional. One has to do with feeling satisfied; the other concerns performance. Being able to "perform"—to have erections when you want them, for example—is certainly important to men. When a man experiences difficulties in performing the way he would like to, he understandably feels upset and wants to do something about it. As important as this may be, however, the ability to perform is only at the periphery of male sexual needs. Although in the past this may have been enough, today men want more from their sexual relationships than the ability to function normally.

For a long time men have been silent about their sexual concerns and unhappiness. Seldom do men share their real feelings about what they get, or don't get but want, from a sexual relationship. Most male "sex talk" is not honest talk at all; problems and concerns are causes of embarrassment, so they get covered up. Dissatisfaction is not voiced because men are not thought of as being sexually sensitive. Instead, our usual view of men is that they are rugged sexual machines, driven by a strong sex instinct, easily aroused, and wanting or needing nothing more than regular orgastic release in order to be satisfied. This myth is at the root of much unhappiness for men and women. Realizing that men are sexually sensitive and that they, too, have sexual needs beyond orgasm is fundamental for undoing many performance problems and moving toward sexual fulfillment.

Although this book is directed mainly at men, it is not my intent to exclude women from my audience. On the contrary, the material presented here concerns women as much as it does men. Sexual fulfillment is not something that can be achieved alone. Whether you are involved with a man who has one steady partner or many partners, true sexual fulfillment concerns *relationships*. It is not possible in any relationship for one partner to be sexually fulfilled while the other is sexually unsatisfied. Overcoming specific sexual difficulties, achieving specific sexual goals (such as learning to delay orgasm), and moving toward sexual fulfillment are goals that are best accomplished when they are pursued by two people working together.

Generally speaking, sexual satisfaction is usually given a low priority in relationships, and this in itself is one reason why so many people complain of difficulties, concerns, and general feelings of sexual discontent. The old phrase "The honeymoon is over" is, unfortunately, often true for couples who have been together for a while. Of course, not only sex is neglected; often couples complain of a lack of intimacy and fun in their lives as well. Many of the exercises in this book are designed to help you reestablish this intimacy and fun as well as promote sexual satisfaction, since all are directly related to one another and to the overall quality of a relationship. Often, it is not just one of these areas that needs some attention, but all three.

This book was written now because I believe that the time is ripe for change. More and more, men and women alike are questioning the *quality* of their lives together. Men are more willing to challenge some of the basic ideas about male sexuality, to take some risks, and to make changes in their lives that will lead them to feeling happier. Changing, however, is almost always a slow process requiring patience and persistence. The ideas we learn as children lead to habits that are difficult to break, even when we want to. Don't expect to be able to change your sexual habits any more easily than you can change any of your other habits. On the other hand, if you are motivated, and if you and your partner have shared goals, this book can help you to achieve them.

The content of this book stems from my experience as a sex therapist, teacher, and researcher. I did not grow up wanting to be a sexologist. I wanted at first to be an accountant, like my father, but ended up becoming an engineer instead. I subsequently changed careers, becoming first a school psychologist, then a clinical psychologist. Eventually, I specialized in the area of human sexuality. Working with men and women unhappy in their relationship or perhaps, experiencing specific performance difficulties, I became privy to this most hidden aspect of ourselves. In the process of helping these couples, I learned as much from them as they learned from me. In this book I am attempting to share what I have learned.

Though this is an original work, I, like most writers, am

indebted to the thinking of others. Among those whose ideas have influenced me are Drs. John Gagnon and Donald Mosher. Dr. Gagnon has written about the nature of sexual relationships in our society; his concept of sexual *scripts* has found its way into my thinking as well. Dr. Mosher first introduced me to the idea of sexual *schemas*. He impressed on me the need to look at sexual desire not as something simple that is the same for everyone, but rather as a complex phenomenon that depends on a great many factors.

There are others to whom I am indebted, both for the opportunity to write this book and for its content. From 1977 through 1979 I held a postdoctoral fellowship, sponsored by the National Institute of Mental Health under a grant awarded to Dr. Richard Green. Without that support this book would not have come about. From its beginning my editors, Lynne Lumsden and Don Chanfrau of Spectrum Books, and Dr. Carl Thoresen of Stanford University, were enthusiastic and supportive. During the course of the writing Dr. David Beatty and Leslie LoPiccolo were generous with their time and ideas; there were many instances in which our conversations helped me clarify my thinking and make it more easily understood by others. Drs. Harvey Gochros and Joel Fischer reviewed an early version of the manuscript and provided many helpful comments. Nina Fontana, Vivian Stabiner, and Janet Golding typed, read, proofed, and shared their reactions; their patience and good humor were most helpful. Finally, I want to extend my sincerest thanks and appreciation to my friend, Arthur Dobrin, for the use of his poetry.

1 reassessing male and female sexuality

We all have ideals that we strive for and try to live up to. Ideals are vital; they add meaning to our lives. Without ideals, life quickly loses its excitement and we lose our sense of direction. As important as they are, however, ideals can also make for a lot of human misery. This happens when ideals are either so high that we can never hope to reach them, or when they are inhumane, oppressive, and/or stifling. There are several commonly held ideas concerning sexuality, as well as sexual ideals, that seem to fall into these categories. They contribute directly to the development of sexual dysfunctions, in both men and women, and often play a major role in such problems. In other cases, the same ideas and ideals contribute, if not to actual sexual dysfunctions (erection problems, orgasm problems, and so on), then to a general feeling of unhappiness and dissatisfaction with sex. To reduce their negative effects, we need to take a fresh look at some of these ideas. That is, we need to reassess our thinking about sexuality. This will not be easy—it's never easy, or pleasant, to take stock of ourselves—but the potential benefits are considerable.

THE MALE SEXUAL SCRIPT

For a long time, it has been a popular notion that men have a strong and constant sex drive; in short, an ever-present interest in sex that does not need to be stimulated in any way because it is always there. Most men and women today still believe this to be pretty much true. Although some are willing to concede that men, in ways and at times, can be sensitive and that their sex drive can be influenced by circumstances, the prevailing opinion remains that men are "naturally" more sexual than women and that their sexual interest is much less influenced by circumstances than is a woman's. This view of male sexuality forms, in part, the foundation for the kind of arrangement that characterizes most couples' sexual relationships.

The idea that men are always ready for sex, somewhat like machines that are always turned on, is related to the male generally taking the more active role in a sexual relationship. In the drama of life between the sexes, men have always been cast in the role of the pursuer; this is, in a sense, their *script*. They learn this during late childhood and adolescence, between the ages of nine and fifteen or so. Their sources of information are the adults around them, books, movies, television, and, of course, their peers. The sexual script they learn is just one part of a much larger script that describes how to be a man in general. This larger script is the so-called *male role*. In a nutshell, males learn that they are expected to be strong, brave, competitive, unemotional, aggressive, and dominant if they are to get along in the world of men, and they start at a very early age to develop these traits in themselves. Eventually, they come to feel that it is "natural" for them to be this way and "abnormal" for them to be some other way, for instance, emotional or gentle. The adults and peers in their lives encourage this. Teachers and parents, for example, worry if a boy seems to lack aggressiveness. Their fear reflects a concern that a gentle boy will not make a successful man.

The male *sexual script* calls for a man to be the one who pursues the woman sexually, usually from the beginning of a relationship, and to press for as much sexual contact as he can get. He is encouraged to keep on testing the limits in a relationship. Traditionally, the ultimate sexual goal that men have been encouraged to seek is intercourse, and having intercourse with a woman is taken as a personal accomplishment, an achievement, as well as a pleasurable experience in itself. As a result, boys grow to be men who are preoccupied with genital contact and intercourse and who are relatively uninterested in other forms of sexual contact, such as touching and kissing, which they consider to be second best.

The male sexual script gives the man responsibility for turning on his partner during a sexual encounter. During adolescence, boys learn, largely from other boys, plus books, movies, and television, what sorts of things they should do in order to seduce a girl and get her sexually aroused. This includes information about how to set the stage, so to speak, by choosing the right setting for sex, things to say and do, what to wear, how to look, and so on. They also get some ideas about how and where to kiss and fondle a woman's body in order to get her excited. A lot of this information may be inaccurate, but boys don't know this at the time; they are eager to learn their script.

Because of the role he must play in a sexual encounter, a man must learn to rely mainly on *psychic stimulation* to become sexually aroused himself. He learns, in other words, to focus his attention on his partner's body and her responsiveness to his lovemaking as sources of arousal for him. This is why most men say that doing things to a woman and getting her turned on is a turn-on for them.

By the time they are adults, most males tend to view their own sexual behavior (that is, their script) as natural. They think that they were born to be the pursuers in sexual relationships.

Actually, the sexual script men live by is largely learned. This is evident when you read about sexual behavior in other cultures, where people learn other scripts. There are places in the world, for instance, where men are raised to be passive and sensitive, while women are taught aggressiveness. These cultures also have their sexual scripts, but they are different from the ones we live by. Probably people in all cultures view their own sexual behavior and scripts in the same way—as natural rather than learned. When you consider how young we are when we begin to develop our sex roles and sexual scripts, it is not surprising that it might be difficult later on to view them as anything other than nature's way. However, it is important for you now to try thinking in terms of learning rather than nature. If you can learn one sexual script, you can learn others.

THE FEMALE SEXUAL SCRIPT

At the same time that the man in a relationship is playing the part of the pursuer and the actively sexual person, the woman's script reflects a different but complementary role. The female sexual script, like its counterpart in men, reflects traditional thinking about the "nature" of female sexuality.

Until very recently, people who wrote books like this one, about how to have a better sex life, presented a view of women as much less sexual than men. Their idea was that a woman had only latent sexual interests. They believed that, if left alone, a woman would never spontaneously think about sex or feel "horny." All her sexual feelings were thought to be dormant, or sleeping.

The sexual script that emerges from the above notions about women's sexuality is essentially a passive one. According to myth, it is only the man who is skillful at lovemaking, and who perhaps loves her, who can "awaken" a woman's sex drive. Therefore, the woman's role in a sexual relationship becomes a much less active one than the man's. She does, of course, make a contribution to the sexual relationship, and she too learns how to do this during later childhood and adolescence. Probably the most important part of the female's sexual script is to be sexually desirable. She accomplishes this through the way she looks, the way she acts toward a man, and the things she says to him. If she is interested in sexual contact or a relationship with him, she can encourage a man's initiative, but she must do this in a way that lets the major responsibility remain with him. She may, for instance, provide a romantic setting, dress in ways she knows he likes, compliment him, and so on. In comparison to the man's role, her role is much more subtle and requires a great deal of sensitivity and skill. For this reason, women are considered seductive and clever. Their sexual script also mainly concerns the stages prior to an actual sexual encounter, what might be called the *prelude*. During a typical actual sexual encounter between a man and a woman, however, the woman is usually much more passive. Her sexual arousal comes mainly from *direct stimulation*—the things her lover does to her body.

In addition to being less active and more subtle, the female sexual script requires that a woman more or less guard her body. For a long time, married women were legally considered to be the property of their husbands, and they were regarded as guilty of a crime (or sin) if they had relations with (or sexual feelings for) other men. Among unmarried women, virginity prior to marriage was held up as a great virtue, partially for the same reason. A nonvirgin was considered to be tainted property and an outcast. As one reflection of this, the female sexual script demands that a woman learn to control not only her own sexual feelings but also those of men. She needs to be able to maintain a man's interest in her, while still setting some limits on his actual sexual behavior.

The male and female sexual scripts seem to be undergoing change in recent years. There is some recognition, as we have said, that men can be sensitive. Also, women are now credited with having a sex drive and are freer today to take the initiative.

However, personal research and experience in therapy indicate that the traditional sexual arrangement, which is characterized by the sexual scripts already described, is still going strong. Among the majority of couples who are married or living together in a maritallike arrangement, sexual scripts are the rule rather than the exception.

SEXUAL SCRIPTS AND SEXUAL DYSFUNCTIONS

The sexual scripts described in the previous sections not only can interfere with a couple's sexual pleasure, but they can also contribute directly to sexual dysfunctions in both men and women.

The first problem with traditional thinking about male sexuality is that it really is dehumanizing. The idea that men are always interested in sex reduces them to the level of rabbits—or worse, since even a rabbit's sex drive takes breaks! Men are not sexual machines, but if we encourage them to think that way, they will end up making love like machines. Thinking that they are sexually insensitive, and should perform like machines, also makes it more likely that men will experience sexual difficulties when they try to live up to this image. A number of men actually feel there is something wrong with them because they are not always interested in sex or because they don't always perform at the same level. Others may not feel "abnormal" because they do not always want sex or do not perform equally well, but they don't exactly feel comfortable about it either. Almost all men find it embarrassing to tell a woman, "No thanks, I'm not interested right now"; they fear that a woman will think less of them for having such feelings. Similarly, few men can experience, say, problems getting an erection and still enjoy a sexual encounter. They usually feel intense shame when they have such an experience and it usually ruins the encounter for them.

The idea that men are constantly sexual implies that they are not sensitive, at least not sexually sensitive. While much attention has been paid to women's sexual delicacy and their needs to be treated in certain ways and have certain conditions met in order to feel sexually turned on, very little attention has been given to men's needs in these areas. Most people believe that men are sexually rugged, and they are surprised when a man's sensitivities show up in the form of a sexual dysfunction.

>Mr. X, age eighteen, called me in a state of near panic. He had a sexual problem, he said, and had to speak to me about it as soon as possible. When he arrived at my office the next morning, it was apparent that he was still very much upset. Sitting on the edge of his chair, he told me the following story:

>He and his girlfriend, whom he had been seeing steadily for about two years, had been thinking about getting engaged. Although he was quite attractive and had had a number of girlfriends, Mr. X was somewhat shy and had never, before the time he was about to describe, gone beyond the level of kissing and petting during a sexual encounter. However, one night the weekend before, he and his girlfriend went to a movie. The film was a romantic story about a young couple with whom they obviously could identify. The movie included a scene in which the young couple go to bed together for the first time. Mr. X fondled his girl a little during the film, and once or twice they kissed. Her reactions that night, however, were different from usual. At one point, for instance, she took his hand and put it on her thigh, something she had never done before. He found that both exciting and a bit scary, since he was conscious of being in a crowded theater.

>After the movie ended, they walked to his car, where Mr. X discovered that his girlfriend was still very much turned on. They kissed passionately, and this time she placed his hand on her breast. He found that very exciting, too, but not nearly so exciting as the strokes she began to give his genitals through his pants. As they continued to pet, Mr. X was both turned on and, by his own admission, more than a little nervous. He was very

aware of being in a lighted parking lot, with cars on either side, and felt very vulnerable. As their petting intensified, he found himself very aroused by his girl's passion, but still nervous about the situation. As he unbuttoned her blouse, for example, he found himself looking around for police cars, and when they laid down on the seat and he caressed her genitals through her pants, he kept worrying about being discovered. Then, suddenly, his girlfriend said to him, "Let's do it. I'm ready. Let's do it now."

Although he had dreamed about just such a moment, at the time all Mr. X could think of was the fact that he was in the middle of that parking lot. He kept thinking about the police. He tried to put the thoughts out of his mind as he awkwardly removed his girlfriend's pants. Then, glancing around all the time, he tried to pull his own pants down without doing anything that might attract attention. When he did this he found, to his surprise, that his penis was not erect. He was shocked. Usually, he was erect almost all the time, sometimes uncomfortably so, when he and his girl would make out. But now, when he seemed finally to have a use for it, the damned thing was flaccid. Then his girlfriend took a peek, saw that he didn't have an erection, and started to cry. At that point, Mr. X was so upset he didn't know what to do. He couldn't even talk. He pulled up his pants, turned on the ignition, and drove out of the parking lot. After a while, his girlfriend stopped crying, but they rode all the way to her house in silence.

Young Mr. X's experience is not really unusual, nor are his reactions or those of his girlfriend. Both were following their respective sexual scripts, and both got trapped by them. Obviously, Mr. X's sexuality was more sensitive than either he or his partner thought it should be, and what might otherwise have been simply a frustrating experience ended up being a crisis in their relationship. At the time we spoke, Mr. X felt that there was something very wrong with him, and he was afraid to face his girlfriend again, much less try a second sexual encounter.

Mr. Y was in his midforties and had always been single. In recent years, he had been experiencing erection problems intermittently, especially the first few times he went to bed with a woman, and he came to see me to find out if there was something that could be done about it. At one point, he related the following incident. It illustrates quite clearly the problems involved in breaking away from the male sexual script.

> Mr. Y was in a bar-restaurant near his home having a late dinner by himself. At that hour, the place was fairly crowded, and the customers included several women who were either eating or drinking alone. It was a small, cozy restaurant, and it also was a popular bar among local singles who were over thirty. Mr. Y had met a couple of women there, but he really preferred just to eat there on occasion. On this particular night he noticed, as he was eating, that one woman at the bar would occasionally look his way. Once, twice, then three times their eyes met. He thought she was interested in him and that she was attractive, but after flirting with a fourth glance, he finally decided he really wasn't interested that night, and he didn't look her way anymore.
>
> Mr. Y finished his dinner and was about to leave when he caught sight of the woman again, out of the corner of his eye, staring at him. He looked her way, and she caught his eye with an intense stare. Then, to his chagrin, she got down from her stool and started toward him. She didn't have to go too far for him to see that she was more than a little drunk, and he felt himself tense up as she got closer. She did just what he was afraid she would do, which was to sit down beside him and begin flirting in a very obviously sexual manner. Mr. Y was embarrassed by and uncomfortable with her come-on, which was much too strong for him. Also, although the woman was definitely attractive, he really was not at that point interested in pursuing the opportunity she was offering. He knew quite well that she was not the sort of woman he felt comfortable with, and he had reason, based on past experience, to expect that he would have trouble getting an erection if he went to bed with her.
>
> Mr. Y tried to handle the situation as best he could. First, he tried to turn the encounter into a conversation; then, he tried humoring her; finally, he just tried to escape as gracefully as

possible. To do this, he told the woman he was leaving town on business that same night, would have liked to spend more time with her, but simply couldn't. He asked for her phone number and promised he would call her when he got back from his "trip."

Mr. Y's experience may strike you as familiar. Obviously, the problem of dealing with someone who likes you, but in whom you are not interested at the moment, is common for both men and women. However, it perhaps is a bit more of a bind for men than women. Because it is consistent with her sexual script, a woman can refuse a man's offer of sexual contact without any feeling of shame. She is *expected* to guard her body and will be respected for not offering it up to just anyone. However, it is not part of a man's sexual script to refuse an offer of sexual contact from a woman. After all, he is supposed to be always up for sex. Therefore, most men experience at least a twinge of shame if and when they actually turn down such an offer, especially if it comes from a woman whom most people would regard as attractive. Generally speaking, it is not something they are proud of and enjoy talking about. This was certainly true in Mr. Y's case, for he was evidently embarrassed when he related the above story. I told him that what he had done sounded good to me—the fact that he did avoid a sexual encounter in that situation was a sign that he was beginning to learn what was good for him and to act on that knowledge. It was a sign that he was beginning to appreciate his own sexual needs and sensitivities.

My reaction evoked first a sigh of relief, and then a large grin from Mr. Y. He told me that had been the first time he had ever turned down a woman's offer of sex and that he had felt very uncomfortable about it. He really didn't know, he said, if he had done the right thing. He then related several other incidents—times when he had found himself in rather uncomfortable positions or, as he put it, "hanging from the ceiling by my thumbs, trying to grin and like it." He seldom functioned well sexually under such circumstances, and neither would I.

Both Mr. X's actual sexual dysfunction and Mr. Y's potential one were related in a very direct way to the fact that neither had ever spent much time thinking about what they didn't want. Neither had ever considered the possibility that they had sexual sensitivities; in short, that their sexual performance was affected by circumstances. Instead, both believed in the myth that men are sexual machines, and they ended up expecting too much from themselves as human beings. As typical men, they were prone to letting themselves get caught up in situations that were not conducive to their own sexual needs, and their performances suffered for it. Of the two, Mr. Y was closer to helping himself, in that he was beginning to assert himself sexually, in this case by avoiding a situation he was not attracted to and which he knew was likely to lead to sexual performance problems. He had not as yet, however, taken the positive step of discovering what he did want in terms of a sexual partner, the right situation, and so on, and actively seeking it out.

The first way in which sexual scripts contribute to sexual dysfunction in men, then, is related to the fact that the male sexual script leads men to expect too much of themselves. By regarding ourselves as sexual machines, we men neglect our sensitivities and end up in situations that are not conducive to good sexual performance. Ironically, we then think that there is something wrong with us sexually, when in fact what is really wrong is our thinking about ourselves.

A second way in which following their sexual script sets the stage for sexual dysfunctions in men is that it turns every sexual encounter into a performance. Because the script gives them responsibility for getting both themselves and their partners turned on, the situation becomes one in which they can either "fail" or "succeed" in accomplishing this goal. Worrying about success versus failure in any situation (sexual or otherwise) is called *performance anxiety*. Since anxiety (nervous tension) is known to interfere with sexual performance, the sexual script that men follow sets them up in a very real sense to have problems as they start worrying more and more about how well they are going to perform in bed.

Mr. A's situation was in many ways typical of the sort of position in which men often find themselves. Recently divorced, in his middle thirties, Mr. A had become, after twelve relatively sheltered years, a member of the growing singles culture. As he described it, this scene is both exciting and threatening; a way of life that is very competitive, often lonely, and in which lasting relationships seem few and far between.

> During his marriage Mr. A had rarely experienced any sexual difficulties, although he had found that his interest in sex dropped off some over time. Otherwise, he had only the occasional problem with getting or keeping an erection that virtually all men experience now and then. Since becoming single, however, he had been having sexual problems regularly. These difficulties tended to concern mostly his ability to maintain an erection during a sexual encounter, although occasionally he had trouble even getting an erection.

> Mr. A experienced women in general as having changed a lot during the twelve years he had been married. This impression was encouraged, to say the least, by articles he read in different "men's magazines." To sum it up, he had come to believe that: women expected to go to bed with a man on their first date if they liked him; women expected to have at least one and preferably several orgasms during each and every sexual encounter; women expected a man's erection to last as long as necessary for them to reach orgasm; and, finally, women wanted their sexual encounters to include a lot of creative foreplay and afterplay. The men's magazines that Mr. A read were full of helpful hints on how to accomplish these things; in other words, on how to make himself into a superlover whose technique could knock the socks off any woman who got into bed with him.

Because of his belief about what was expected of him, Mr. A approached women with a good deal of uneasiness. He was afraid that he would not be able to handle all of the expectations he thought a modern, liberated woman would have. It took him some time to overcome these worries and start dating. When he did finally start dating and went to bed with women, he found that he was sometimes unable to get an erection, and at other times that he would get one, but lose it soon after penetration. Understandably, he was very upset.

Performance anxiety is almost inescapable for men in our culture. The male sexual script, with its emphasis on the man having the responsibility for arousing both himself and his partner during a sexual encounter, creates a situation in which the man simply has to be concerned with his performance. The case of Mr. A is, then, far from the exception. He got trapped precisely because he followed the pattern that has been laid out for men in their sexual relationships with women. By worrying so much about whether he was capable of fulfilling the responsibilities he thought were his, he ended up not being able to function at all. This pattern seems to be changing, but slowly. In the interim, the fact that women are expecting more from their sexual relationships only seems to increase performance anxiety among men who feel that it is their responsibility alone to meet all of these expectations. The answer is not for women to want less, but for men and women to liberate themselves from oppressive sexual scripts.

The male sexual script also makes men vulnerable to sexual dysfunctions in that it encourages them to rely on psychic stimulation as their main source of sexual arousal. By being the more active one in a sexual encounter—the "doer"—the traditional sexual arrangement followed by couples in our culture leads to the man being turned on mainly by his partner's physical appearance, plus her responsiveness to what he does to her when they make love. In other words, the way her body looks, plus the way she groans, moans, tosses, and turns in response to him, is a turn-on for the man. There is no doubt that this can be very arousing indeed. However, this arrangement also leaves men in a position of not developing (or developing very little) other possible ways of getting aroused, especially through direct stimulation. For instance, while all men are aware that the glans of the penis is an erogenous zone, few men have the same sort of appreciation for their other erogenous zones that women do. Few people would argue that men in general do not think of themselves as sensual. Rather than developing the erotic potential of their bodies as a whole, they are inclined instead to concentrate more or less exclusively on their penises. One of the reasons for this is perhaps the fact that their traditional role in sexual encounters does not lend itself to their developing as much of a sense of their physical sensuality as it could. In fact, it can be argued that their script keeps men focused on their genitals to the exclusion of the rest of their bodies.

As a man ages, he may require more stimulation to become sexually aroused to the point of having an erection. Obviously, it is in his interest, then, to develop and use as many channels of sexual arousal as possible, both direct and psychic. Inasmuch as sticking to a sexual script prevents him from getting as much direct stimulation (of his body by his partner) as he might, that script can contribute to his having a sexual dysfunction. Many middle-aged and older men find themselves in this very position; they have become channeled by their limiting sexual script in such a way that they do not get the stimulation they need in order to become sexually aroused.

Just as the male sexual script limits men, the female sexual script limits women to narrow, inflexible roles in their sexual encounters with men. The female sexual script, therefore, contributes to sexual frustration and dysfunctions in women, just as the male sexual script contributes to such problems in men. As discussed earlier, the sexual arrangement that has been encouraged and practiced by most couples has given the man virtually all the responsibility for the outcome of a sexual encounter, while the woman has next to none. She does have a role to play, of course, in enticing a man to desire her sexually, and she probably feels some responsibility to please him, but by and large the sexual encounter is the man's show. Evidence of this is easy to find. Popular songs and poems about lovemaking compare the man to an artist or musician, while the woman is his inspiration, his canvas, or his instrument. This same theme is repeated in countless romantic novels.

A woman may very well want to be inspiring (sexy) and a good "instrument" (responsive), but her role in the sexual encounter is not at all like the man's. She is limited by her script to being the one who reacts rather than initiates, who responds rather than directs. By following her script, therefore, the woman cannot avoid a certain feeling of helplessness in sexual situations, just as the man cannot escape his feelings of responsibility. She may be bothered by this a lot or not at all, but that is not really the point. What is important is that her role limits the woman's ability to get what she wants. Because she has less freedom to take the initiative, a woman who follows her sexual script must depend on her partner's skill and initiative for her sexual fulfillment. There are several reasons why this may be unsatisfactory, the first of which is that men are not born with lovemaking skills any more than they are born with woodworking skills. Men have to develop their lovemaking skills, and the way they do this is through reading and talking with other men, and through plain old trial-and-error experience. While they are learning, their partners must put up with their lack of sexual skill. Since many women say that a man younger than thirty years of age seldom knows much about lovemaking, we are talking about a lot of waiting. By the time their partners become sexually skillful, many women may have lost interest in sex.

A second problem with making love according to the script is that it does not allow for spontaneity except as initiated by the man. It makes sense that a woman would not always want to do the same sorts of things, sexually, any more than she would always want to hear the same sort of music. However, although she may know what she would like to do at a given moment, her sexual script requires a woman to wait passively and hope that her lover somehow divines her desire. If he doesn't, which is likely since men can't read minds, she is apt to feel frustrated and angry with him. Being dependent on her lover's sexual skills, and having to rely on him to know what she would like, often leaves a woman in a position of not getting what she wants in a sexual encounter. It is no wonder, then, considering these limitations, that women so frequently complain of not feeling aroused during their sexual encounters and of losing their interest in sex.

The female sexual script, like the male's, creates a situation in which women do not have an opportunity to develop fully their potential for becoming sexually aroused. Their limitation is just the opposite of men's. Under the arrangement that calls for the man to be the active one, a woman has little choice but to focus predominantly on the feelings she gets when her partner stimulates her body (direct stimulation). The woman's position, then, is complementary to the man's. In a traditional sexual encounter, each partner is limited to one main source, or channel, of sexual arousal, while the other remains largely undeveloped. In the woman's case, the developed channel is the direct one; in the man's, it is the psychic. The man will be fortunate if his lover is attractive to him and responds to his lovemaking in ways that he likes. Under these conditions, he will get turned on. The woman will get turned on if it happens that her lover does things to her that do please her, but if he doesn't, she is stuck. Because she is not free to switch places, to make love to the man and get aroused by a psychic stimulation (his appearance plus his responsiveness to her), or even to tell him what she wants (for fear he will think her too aggressive), she may not be able to experience very much sexual arousal, and certainly not enough to reach orgasm.

The image of the traditional sexual arrangement between a

man and a woman that is depicted by the sexual scripts described here may seem exaggerated. Some readers may argue that neither men nor women are as limited in their lovemaking as the scripts suggest. For some couples, this is true, and if they have broken free of their sexual scripts, they are indeed fortunate. Presently however, these people are a minority, and most couples still pattern their sexual relationships pretty much according to the scripts described. As a consequence, they make themselves vulnerable to sexual dysfunctions. They also lay themselves open, in the long run, to feelings of boredom, disappointment, and a general sense of being sexually unfulfilled. Few relationships can tolerate such feelings, in one partner or both, for very long.

BEING FUNCTIONAL VERSUS BEING FULFILLED

Perhaps the most common sexual problem that couples face today is not so much a specific sexual *dysfunction* (difficulty with erection, inability to reach orgasm, and others), as a general feeling of *dissatisfaction* with their sexual relationship. So often by the time a couple has been together for a few years, the hopes and expectations each had for what two people could get from a sexual relationship have given way to disappointment, bitterness, sometimes even open hostility. Partners may blame themselves and become depressed, or they may lay blame for their unhappiness on the other's "sexual inadequacy." Either way, the relationship suffers.

It would be grossly oversimplifying and underestimating the difficulties of maintaining a relationship today to suggest that sexual scripts are the sole cause for the sort of situation described above. However, they are one of the prime causes for the sort of sexual dissatisfaction that people complain of more and more. The great majority of these people do not have sexual dysfunctions, that is, they are not men who have trouble getting erections or ejaculating too quickly, or women who don't experience orgasm. What they are suffering from is, in a way, much more complex, and therefore more difficult to deal with, than a sexual dysfunction; it is a feeling of not being sexually fulfilled. They feel frustrated and often turned off to sex. To make up for this, they may look for other things in their relationship that might fill the gap. Sometimes this works and a couple is happy even though they don't get a lot out of their sexual relationship. Then, too, people sometimes do find other things, besides sex, that fill their need for personal fulfillment. Unfortunately, these things may lay outside of the relationship—for example, a job—and therefore do little to bring a couple closer. The most common response to feeling sexually unfulfilled is to continue seeking fulfillment, but with a different partner. Obviously, this too places the relationship at risk.

There probably are no more people today who feel sexually unfulfilled than there were, say, 50 or 100 years ago. It is more likely that people simply feel freer today to express their sexual dissatisfaction. In days when men, and especially women, expected very little from sex, getting very little was no surprise. Complaining, in 1910, that you felt sexually unfulfilled would not draw you much sympathy. It would be like complaining about the weather: everyone does it, but no one really expects anything to change. Also, before the advent of modern birth control methods people had very good reason to fear sex and therefore to avoid it. Since the beginning of this century, however, much progress has been made in liberating sex from reproduction. The development of effective and inexpensive means of birth control has meant that people have become freer to pursue the pleasures of a sexual relationship without fear of pregnancy. Given this opportunity, they have done what you might expect, which is to take advantage of it. Because of the power of sexual pleasure, moreover, they have gradually come to want and expect more and more from the sexual aspect of their relationship.

What people want, today, is not simply to be *functional* (to remain free from a sexual dysfunction), but to feel sexually *fulfilled*. This is becoming true, more and more, for men as well as for women. And this is contrary to the traditional view of men, which would have us believe that a man will be satisfied with his sexual relationship as long as he can get an erection and have an orgasm, preferably through intercourse, as often as he wants. In short, most people have believed that all a man wants out of a sexual relationship is to be able to screw as often as he can. As long as he can "get it up" and "get off," it has been assumed that a man will be happy. Yet—and this may be surprising to some—a number of men who are functional and who do have sex regularly still feel that there is something missing from their sex lives. Somehow, despite the fact that they can perform without difficulty, they feel unhappy and dissatisfied. What some of these men want may, of course, be impossible to achieve. In most cases, however, their expectations are not unreasonable. True, they are dreamers, but what these men (and women) want is for the most part obtainable. It does require making some basic changes in their sexual relationships, though.

One of the keys to sexual fulfillment is being able to break away from the sexual scripts we learn as adolescents and to begin rebuilding our sexual relationships on the basis of a different set of assumptions about the way men and women are sexually. Making love according to the sexual scripts can be exciting. It is fun for a man to pursue a woman, to be turned on by her body, to enjoy doing things to her, and to experience her responsiveness to him. Women say that it is also fun to be pursued, to be made love to by someone who is interested in them. The problem is not so much with this pattern of lovemaking in itself, but in the fact that it tends to become the *only* pattern that couples follow, time after time after time. Because of the nature of the scripts themselves, it is difficult to see how couples would not in the long run find this arrangement boring, frustrating, or both. It is little wonder that so many people are less than enthusiastic about sex, and why a good number of them would just as soon watch television or go to sleep. For many men who are stuck within their sexual script, the only excitement they might get is from making love to a new partner—to be turned on by a new body and a different way of responding—or, by turning their sex lives into an arena for achievement, trying to make it with as many women as possible.

To free ourselves from the need to limit our lovemaking to a single pattern, it would be helpful if we could reassess some of our ideas about male and female sexuality. We need to give some serious thought to questions like the following:

- Are men really more aggressive and interested in sex because they are born that way, or because they are encouraged to be that way, in fact, because they are told there would be something wrong with them if they weren't?
- Are men really "naturally" insensitive and rough, or have they not been encouraged to develop their sensitivity and a capacity for gentleness?
- Are men naturally less sensual, less aware of the erotic potential of their own bodies than women are, or has their sexual script stood in the way of their developing such an awareness?
- Are men preoccupied with intercourse as the be-all and end-all of sex because that is the way they are made, or because the traditional sexual arrangement has made sex a performance and intercourse an accomplishment for them?
- Are women "naturally" less interested in sex, less sexually aggressive than men, or do they act that way because their sexuality has been suppressed, because they have been told that it would be wrong for them to be more sexual?
- Are women "naturally" more difficult to arouse sexually than men, more delicate than men are, or are they limited by virtue of being dependent, because of their sexual script, on a man's initiative and lovemaking skills?

This is not to say that some *natural* differences do not exist between men and women—differences in sexual behavior and in some preferences that we are born with, rather than learn.

However, the traditional views of male and female sexuality exaggerate these differences, and they are oversimplified and unnecessarily restrictive. The ideas on which the male and female sexual scripts are based sell us short, both men and women alike. They need to be challenged if we are to realize the potential that our sexual relationships have within them. We need to consider two alternative possibilities. The first is that men are really more sexually sensitive than has previously been acknowledged. In line with this, we need to consider the possibility that men have the potential to develop their sensuality well beyond the level they usually do. The second idea is that women are really more sexual than they have been given credit for. As one woman colleague put it, "Women get turned on all the time and it seems silly to pretend otherwise." Agreed; we do need to stop pretending. We need to accept the idea that women have a sex drive just as men do. More than that, women are just as capable as men of acting on that sex drive, of taking the initiative and getting pleasure from being the active one, the "doer," in a sexual encounter.

Another way to look at the changes we need to make is to start with the idea that men and women are equally capable of experiencing sexual pleasure and arousal through *both* direct and psychic stimulation. The only reason why men have been channeled into relying on psychic stimulation, and women on direct stimulation, is the sexual script they follow when making love. By clinging to these scripts, neither sex has an opportunity to develop their full potential for erotic pleasure. Men cannot learn to appreciate the erotic potential of their bodies if they must always be the active ones in their sexual encounters, that is, if they never get a chance to be the one who is made love to. Women cannot experience the erotic power that can come from someone else's responses if they never get a chance to be the lover in a sexual encounter.

To accomplish the above, we do not necessarily need to throw away our sexual scripts, but we do need to liberate ourselves from following them exclusively. Making love in the traditional way, as we have said, can most definitely be a delightful experience for both partners. However, it is only one pattern for lovemaking. For men and women to develop their full sexual potential, they need to be able to make love according to other patterns, especially the pattern in which the woman becomes the active one and makes love to her man, and to make up new patterns for themselves. In place of rigidity, then, sexual fulfillment requires flexibility and a willingness at times to give responsibility and control to the other person.

If we are to achieve the sort of flexibility that is needed to experience a greater sense of sexual fulfillment, we must shift the burden of responsibility for what happens in a sexual encounter from the man alone to the man and the woman together. The man, in other words, needs to give up some control, and the woman needs to accept some. Having all of the responsibility for the outcome of a sexual encounter may make men feel powerful and competent, at least if they succeed in getting their partners turned on and bringing themselves and their women to orgasm. But responsibility also means pressure. Since nobody likes to fail or to seem incompetent, men seek praise for their lovemaking abilities, hide their ignorance, and all too often get upset at the slightest hint of criticism. And this does nothing to help the woman, who feels hesitant to utter anything but praise for fear it will crush her lover to hear that he is somewhat less than perfect.

By following the traditional sexual arrangement, the sexual encounter becomes more than a shared experience of pleasure and intimacy; it becomes a real performance in which the man can either succeed or fail. Most men, if they think about it, are aware of this. They report that they seldom are able to escape being self-conscious—watching themselves perform during a sexual encounter. If things happen to go poorly, it is their failure; if they go well, it is their achievement. This is very different from the way things would be if the man and the woman shared responsibility equally for their own and one another's sexual pleasure. Under these circumstances, men could stop being self-conscious at times—when they hand control over to the partner—and just enjoy what is happening to them. In addition, a pleasurable sexual encounter is something that would be a credit to the relationship, not to the man alone. It would be something shared. By the same token, an unsatisfying sexual relationship, or a sexual dysfunction, would be a problem that the couple, as a couple, would need to confront and work on together to overcome. Experience in working with couples is convincing proof that this sort of attitude is much more likely to lead to success in relieving a dysfunction than is the view that the man (or the woman) is inadequate and in need of help.

It makes much more sense to think of sexual fulfillment as something to which both partners contribute than to think of it as either the man's or the woman's responsibility. It makes sense to think of sexual dysfunction in this way, too; in fact, that is the way sex therapists go about helping people who have such dysfunctions. Few people, after all, are sexually dysfunctional when they are *alone,* pleasuring themselves. Also, sexual dysfunctions are usually easily cured in a context of self-pleasure (women can learn to give themselves orgasm fairly quickly, as men can learn to delay ejaculation, during masturbation). The real problems, when they exist, usually enter the picture when a couple wants to function well *together.* In this context, both partners have important roles to play if a sexual dysfunction is to be overcome. The same thing applies to sexual fulfillment—it is something to which both partners must contribute if it is to happen. It is only an illusion to believe that, in a relationship, true sexual fulfillment can exist for one partner but not the other. The person who is feeling unfulfilled—unhappy, dissatisfied—will never be able to give freely to the other, and so both will be frustrated in the long run.

To say that sexual fulfillment is best pursued together does not mean that you as an individual man cannot do things to help yourself develop your sexual potential. There are many ways in which you can grow personally that have little to do with your partner. Many of the exercises in this book are designed to facilitate your personal growth and development as an individual. However, there are limitations on how much you can realize sexual fulfillment all by yourself, and this is where your relationship becomes important. If you have a partner who also wants to seek sexual fulfillment, for herself as well as you, then the changes you make in yourself, plus your cooperative efforts together, will be your means of getting there.

Laying responsibility for sexual satisfaction on a couple rather than an individual means changing the nature of your relationship in several ways. It means, to begin with, taking a cooperative attitude in which you are willing to be flexible in determining what goes on between the two of you. You as a man can no longer be totally, and always, in control of the situation; sometimes your partner will need to be in control. It also means that you will have to learn to communicate effectively with each other, at least within your sexual relationship. You will need to be able to tell each other, and sometimes show each other, what you want and don't want, what feels good and what doesn't. This will take practice, patience, and a good deal of getting used to. If you succeed, the results will be well worth the effort. The subsequent sections and chapters in this book will be helpful in guiding you through these changes, but the motivation and interest must come from you.

We live in times of change, when people's desire to get more from their sexual relationships is not only exciting, but also threatening. To a greater or lesser extent, most people today (and probably all who read this book) experience concern over their sexual performance. Wanting more out of life, sexually or otherwise, can easily turn from something good into something that is self-destructive. In this case it can be destructive, to you and your relationship, if your desire for sexual fulfillment were to become a source of pressure. Competing, either against yourself or your partner, to become a better lover or to see who is the better lover will surely take the joy out of lovemaking. To turn your desire for a better sex life into just another performance, in which you are self-conscious and give yourself grades during and after each encounter, will undermine your efforts to achieve a sense of sexual fulfillment. If you do that, you really will not have been liberated from the male sexual script at all. Worse, the anxiety you experience over trying to become a superlover may very well lead you (or your partner) towards sexual dysfunction. The key to successful pursuit of sexual fulfillment is precisely the opposite: to reject the male sexual script and its notion that you are totally responsible and need to be a superlover, and to move instead toward viewing sex as a shared experience, between equals, each participant equally responsible for its quality.

A fear that people often express these days concerns the implications of becoming a more sexual person. Men and women express worries; they fear they may become "promiscuous," "degenerate," or "oversexed." It is only natural that we have such fears, given the fact that our sexuality has been portrayed as something that needs to be controlled, therefore, something that is dangerous. To be sure, there are risks involved in using a book such as this one. These risks are greatest if you are in a relationship and want to make changes that your partner does not want you to make. The same risks exist, however, whether you read a book on sexuality or a book, say, on how to become more assertive. If you wanted to be more assertive, but your partner did not want you to be, then certainly you would be taking a risk if you pursued your goal, whether through reading a book, taking a course, or whatever. Similarly, your desire for a more satisfying sex life may run contrary to your partner's wishes. The basic dilemma confronting a person in both these cases is whether they should put their own needs and personal goals above those of their partner, or vice versa. How much are you willing to risk, in other words, to get what you want and to be what you want? No author or book can tell you that. However, if you are in a relationship, give some thought to whether your goals are shared by your partner. Read this book together, not alone. Share your concerns and fears with one another. If it turns out that your goals do conflict, you would be wise to talk about this and try to resolve it. As for fears of becoming a "sex fiend" as a result of reading a book (which boils down to a fear that you will not be able to control your own sexuality), it simply is not true. You will always have the power of choice; therefore you will always have responsibility for your own life. You can indeed become a more sexual and sensual person, but you need not ever lose control of yourself.

SEXUAL MYTHS: IDEALS NOT TO LIVE BY

As mentioned at the beginning of this chapter, we all have ideals that we strive for. These ideals are not to be taken lightly; they are the basis for meaning in our lives. It was also said, however, that ideals can also be the cause of a lot of suffering and unhappiness. When they are so unrealistic that virtually no one can reach them, ideals cause people to lead lives of frustration. When they cause us to limit ourselves rather than realize our potential, they also lead to frustration.

We have ideals with respect to relationships and sex as much as we do in other areas in our lives. There are several commonly held sexual ideals that seem to fall into the category of causing more misery than they are worth. Let's review them now, and you can see if you, too, have been one of their victims.

Sexual Myth 1: Simultaneous Orgasm Means True Love

A romantic notion of the twentieth century is that when two people are truly in love with each other, they will reach orgasm at the same time during intercourse. By this thinking, if a couple doesn't experience simultaneous orgasm, through intercourse, then it isn't true love they feel for one another. In this way, the ability to have simultaneous orgasm becomes a test of a relationship.

This ideal is clearly expressed in the novel *Lady Chatterley's Lover* by D.H. Lawrence, and there are hundreds of other books that advocate the same view. Written in 1928, Lawrence's book caught people's attention partly because it portrayed a woman who was capable of experiencing intense sexual feelings. Before then, the popular view had been that women were asexual—incapable of experiencing much sexual pleasure. Most women apparently believed this and, therefore, did not regard sex as a very important part of their lives. If they did not enjoy sex, they simply thought they were normal. Those few women who may have wanted more from sex would have been regarded as crazy for thinking this way. In Lawrence's book, however, Lady Chatterley, who was like most women, suddenly discovers true love. More importantly, this discovery centers around the fact that she experiences intense sexual feelings and simultaneous orgasm with her lover. At the time it was written, this book may have been inspiring to men and women who rejected, or wanted to reject, the idea that it was impossible (or wrong) for a woman to have sexual feelings. As liberating as this thinking may have been for some at that time, the ideal embodied by the idea of simultaneous orgasm is one that may be impossible for many people to reach.

This raises some interesting questions. If simultaneous orgasm hardly ever happens, does that mean that true love hardly ever happens? What if you experience simultaneous orgasm one time and not the next; does that mean you are not in love anymore? What do you do if you believe you are in love, but you don't experience simultaneous orgasm?

Reaching orgasm together, during intercourse, does seem to be a rare experience. It is also an exceptionally pleasurable experience. However, it does not have much credibility as a test of your feelings about someone else. Those who still believe in the mystical meaning of simultaneous orgasm, and who strive to reach it, may be setting themselves up for constant frustration. There are better ways than that to decide whether you are in love.

Sexual Myth 2: Coital Orgasm Means Maturity

This is a variation of Sexual Myth 1, and it, too, is based largely on sexual ignorance. Like the first myth, it has its origins in the early part of this century. As the idea that women were asexual began to lose popularity and was replaced by the idea that they could feel sexual pleasure, it wasn't long before people began to wonder if women were indeed capable of having orgasm as men were. Sigmund Freud, among others, argued that they were. Again, this was in its time a liberating notion, but one that ended up being distorted due to ignorance about the female anatomy and sexual response. The problem stems from the fact that it was men, rather than women, who were put in the position of deciding what was "natural" for women.

Freud believed that there were two main erogenous zones on a woman's body, the clitoris and the vagina. Somehow, Freud had come to the conclusion that, as a woman matures, her clitoris becomes less sensitive, while her vagina becomes more sensitive. He never did explain just how this change was supposed to take place; nevertheless, he maintained that in a "mature" woman, orgasm results from stimulation of the vagina by the penis during intercourse (the so-called vaginal orgasm). Women who had orgasms through clitoral stimulation (clitoral orgasm), meanwhile, were branded immature. Today we know that clitoral stimulation is as important to female orgasm as stimulation of the glans is to male orgasm. We also know that intercourse produces both vaginal and clitoral stimulation, but that many women cannot get sufficient clitoral stimulation in this way to reach orgasm. We don't say that a man who needs to have his glans stimulated in order to reach orgasm is "immature." There are, however, people who still cling to Freud's views regarding female orgasm. As a consequence, there are women who feel badly about themselves if they can't reach orgasm through intercourse, or if they need extra stimulation of the clitoris to reach that level of arousal.

> Ms. M was in her early thirties. Two years before she consulted with me, she had left her husband for a number of reasons, one being an unsatisfying sexual relationship. Since then, she had several lovers and, through a couple of these relationships, had gradually learned to feel better about herself, sexually and otherwise. One thing that continued to bother her, however, was the fact that she had never reached orgasm during intercourse. She regarded this as a personal fault, as a sign that there was something wrong with her. She thought that perhaps she was holding back, fearful of giving herself sexually to a man. This upset her because she had recently met a man for whom she had very strong feelings. Sexually, she felt more comfortable with him than any man she had been with, and she found other aspects of their relationship rewarding as well. Although she could experience an orgasm when her lover stimulated her in other ways (using his hand, his mouth, or a vibrator), Ms. M did not experience orgasm during intercourse. At first she thought that this might be a temporary thing—that in time she would be able to come during intercourse. As time passed and this did not happen, she found herself getting anxious before sex, upset afterward, and increasingly preoccupied with her "failure." She became depressed to the point where she began to lose sleep and weight. Finally, she contacted her former therapist, who suggested she consult a sex therapist.

Ms. M was no less mature than the sex therapist, nor was she more afraid than anyone else to give herself to someone. We all are immature in ways, and we all have mixed feelings about giving ourselves. Many women do not experience orgasm at all during intercourse; others can, but only when they get some additional clitoral stimulation, for instance, by a vibrator or their partner's hands. Ms. M was being unnecessarily hard on herself for something that was really normal. It may be unfortunate that she had not been able to experience orgasm during intercourse, but it certainly was not a sign of maladjustment or immaturity.

Freud's mistaken idea that the clitoris was not involved in orgasm in "mature" women led people to think that women who needed clitoral stimulation were not capable of having mature relationships with men. It's easy to see how it became a goal for women to be able to have orgasms, if not simultaneously with their partners, then at least during intercourse and without any additional "immature" clitoral stimulation. By thinking this way, however, women are set up to feel like personal failures, and their relationships can be severely threatened on the basis of an idea founded in sexual ignorance.

Sexual Myth 3: The Best Sex Is Aggressive Sex

Lady Chatterley's Lover contains more than a trace of this myth, too, as do most romantic novels and stories, both old and new. The scenario goes something like this:

> The woman at first says no, resisting the man's advances. He persists, gradually wearing her down. Eventually she yields to his insistent demands. He makes love to her in a violently passionate manner, perhaps even hurting her. This awakens the woman's own sexual desires. She then surrenders to the man and falls madly in love with him forever.

This sort of thinking, popularized in books, movies, and finally television, encourages men to be aggressive and even violent in their sexual approaches to women. They do this because they are under the impression that women want it—that being aggressive will prove their feelings and win the everlasting love of the woman they desire. They are led to believe that when a woman says no, she means yes, and that their goal as men is to overcome a woman's resistance. They honestly believe that this is romantic. Unfortunately, this particular myth has been peddled for so long that many people now believe it is natural, the same way they believe that the sexual scripts we learn are "natural." They are encouraged in their thinking by the fact that many men and women do find descriptions of aggressive sexual encounters, like those written by D.H. Lawrence and those depicted in so many pornographic films, sexually exciting. The question is: Is it really "natural" for sex to be violent, or is violent sex simply an extension of the sexual script we learn as we grow up? Does sex have to be violent in order to be good? More and more people agree that the answer is no. We who believe that good sex can be passionate and intense, but not violent or painful, or who believe that good sex can be gentle, may still be in the minority today, but our numbers are growing. Hopefully, as people begin to liberate themselves from the limitations of sexual scripts and the ideas on which they are based, which encourage men and women to guide their sexual relationships in ways such as described above, myths like this one will fall by the wayside.

Sexual Myth 4: Having a Sexual Dysfunction Means There Is Something Wrong With You or Your Relationship

Yet another popular but wrong notion, advocated particularly in the latter half of this century, is that people who are in a good relationship and who are well adjusted don't experience sexual difficulties. Many psychiatrists, psychologists, and other mental health professionals can be counted among those who advocate this particular myth and they burden their patients with it. They do not do so because they want to mislead, but because they believe the myth themselves. They believe that if two people are mature and if they love one another, neither will ever experience problems in their sexual performance.

If you are one who believes this sexual myth, and you happen to develop a sexual dysfunction, you are faced with two possible explanations: either you are immature or else there is something seriously wrong with your relationship. Neither of these possibilities is very attractive, and either one, if true, would represent a major problem. Of course, it is sometimes true that a sexual dysfunction may have something to do with problems in the relationship, or it may, in a sense, be a matter of maturity, as the following example suggests.

> Mr. and Mrs. W were in their late thirties and had been together for nearly ten years. It was Mr. W's second marriage and Mrs. W's first. When they came to see me, each was complaining of sexual difficulties. Mr. W was having trouble regularly getting an erection during his sexual encounters with his wife. Mrs. W complained of a loss of interest in sex as well as a loss of the ability to experience orgasms. From the moment they started therapy, it was very clear that both of their problems were in part due to the fact that their relationship was not a very good one and that their poor relationship was in turn at least partly a reflection of their immaturity as individuals. Mr. W was an extremely self-centered, vain man who struck me as not yet capable of having a mature relationship with a woman, that is, one in which he would give as much as he got. Similarly, he did not seem up to the role of being a father. He regarded his children mainly as a burden and an interference with his activities. He was a chronic complainer who never felt that he was getting what he deserved out of life and who seldom had a good word to say about anyone else. He married Mrs. W mainly because she seemed committed to him, because she earned a good income, and because she was willing to do many things for him. From the beginning, however, he did not return her investment. He went out a lot and always had at least one girlfriend on the side.
>
> Mrs. W married late and had not had very much experience with men before meeting Mr. W. She had spent most of her life, from adolescence onward, in the role of a "parental child"—an older

child who takes a lot of responsibility for the running of a household and the raising of younger siblings. She did this mostly because her mother was sick, on and off, for many years, but also because she was very shy and not self-confident, and she preferred the security of her role at home to the risks and uncertainties of life in the real world. Actually, it seemed the only reason she did marry was that, first, her father died, and second, her youngest sister got married, which then left Mrs. W completely alone. Mr. W, who presented himself as very needy and demanding, actually fit her needs very well—he was a good replacement for her father and sister—and so it was really no surprise that she should be attracted to him. However, she had never felt that she loved her husband; in fact, she didn't believe she knew what love was, or if it really existed.

As you can see, the marriage of Mr. and Mrs. W was really more like a mother-son than a husband-wife relationship, and in this sense their immaturity contributed to their later unhappiness. Neither of them felt very comfortable giving to the other on an emotional level and therefore the stage was set for constant conflict, which was pretty much the story of their marriage. In their sexual relationship, Mr. W's demands and his self-centeredness gradually turned off his wife, who eventually lost, first, her ability to experience orgasm and, later on, her interest in sex. Her anger over his behavior, combined with her own difficulty in giving freely of herself on an intimate, emotional level, resulted in Mrs. W adopting a frankly hostile attitude toward her husband. She resisted his advances, often rejecting him in a very rude manner. When she did consent to going to bed with him, she was completely unresponsive except to complain that he was "taking too long" to reach orgasm. Eventually, Mr. W developed a problem in getting erections, a difficulty for which his wife had little sympathy.

The case of Mr. and Mrs. W shows that, at times, a sexual dysfunction in one or both partners can be linked to other problems within a relationship and/or the individuals in that relationship. This is *not,* however, always the case.

Mr. and Mrs. Z had been married for nearly two years. They sought out sex therapy for Mr. Z's problem, which had to do with premature ejaculation. He would often reach orgasm as he was about to enter his wife; at other times, he would climax within seconds after entering her. Mr. Z had always had this problem with reaching orgasm quickly. He had also been in therapy for years, dealing with a variety of problems, one of which was the premature ejaculation. His therapy helped him a great deal with the other problems he faced, but it had not helped him at all in the sexual area. Unfortunately, both he and his therapist believed Sexual Myth 4 and felt that Mr. Z's premature ejaculation was really just a symptom, a sign of some other problem in him or the relationship. Mr. Z felt happy with his life and his marriage, but the fact that he continued to suffer from premature ejaculation made him doubt his feelings. When I interviewed them, it seemed to me that their marriage was a good one and that both Mr. and Mrs. Z were well adjusted. I, therefore, suggested that the premature ejaculation had nothing to do with immaturity on Mr. Z's part or with a bad marriage. Instead, we focused on treating the premature ejaculation, using a program much like the one that appears later in this book, and, I might add, it was very successful.

As the last example suggests, jumping to the conclusion that having sexual difficulties is a sign of something more deeply wrong with you or your relationship may be unwarranted. To swallow whole the idea that happy, well-adjusted people never have sexual problems is harmful to your emotional health. There can be many different causes of sexual dysfunction, some of which may concern your relationship and others that do not. It is best to consider all the options and not jump to a conclusion based on preconceived ideas such as Sexual Myth 4.

SUMMARY

The basic idea in this chapter is that couples typically pattern their sexual relationships using certain ground rules they learn as youths. This traditional sexual arrangement is sort of like a play, in which both the man and the woman have parts, or scripts, which they act out. Generally, the man is the more active one (the "doer"), and the woman is more passive (the "receiver"). In and of itself, there is nothing wrong with this particular pattern of lovemaking. However, problems arise when people restrict themselves only to this one pattern. One such problem is that, when it is followed exclusively, this pattern gives the man too much responsibility and control and the woman too little. The man is, therefore, forced to be self-conscious, while the woman is, in many ways, helpless. Neither the man nor the woman is free to develop their sexual potential to the fullest, since their scripts channel them into complementary positions: the man gets turned on mainly through his partner's responses, the woman mainly through having her body touched.

The sexual scripts that form the foundation of most sexual relationships can contribute very directly to sexual dysfunctions in both men and women. They can be harmful to a man because they foster self-consciousness and performance anxiety and because they limit his ability to get turned on by being made love to. They are harmful to a woman because they restrict her freedom to get what she wants and because they limit her ability to get turned on by being the active one in a sexual encounter. Because they limit us artificially, our sexual scripts also lead in the long run to feelings of frustration and disappointment, and frequently to a loss of sexual desire.

Although there will always be a certain percentage of people who, at one time or another, develop a sexual dysfunction, a much more common complaint that couples express is a lack of sexual fulfillment. To be in a position to improve their sexual performance (that is, to overcome a sexual dysfunction), their overall sense of satisfaction, or both, people need to reassess some of the traditional ideas about male and female sexuality and to liberate themselves from the need to pattern their lovemaking in only one way. Men and women need to share the responsibility for the quality of their sexual relationship more, rather than have this rest in the hands of the man alone. Men need to learn to give up some control, and women must be willing to accept some.

Gravity And Ribs

I swear you ask for this:
A fastened heart upon the sheet
Anointing the night with blood drops.
But listen to my secret now:
I want to suck your weight down
And be bound by your gravity and ribs.
Seize me and anoint me
In the aroma of hair and warm honey.
Held between you and the earth
I hear the thunder of wild hooves,
Gather flowers in a thousand streets,
And one sunrise dissolves my prison wall.
ARTHUR DOBRIN

2 self-discovery

An incident occurred during an adult education class in male sexuality that a friend and I were leading. It was one of the first times that I talked to a group of men about sexual scripts (as discussed in chapter 1) as a basis for sexual relationships and about their limitations. The men seemed to relate well to what I was saying about the nature of these scripts, the assumptions about male and female sexuality on which they are based, and the problems that they can cause. Naturally, I was pleased. Then, the man sitting beside me, a very pleasant, middle-aged fellow, turned and said, "I think you're right, Joe. I agree with everything you've said. Following those scripts has been the story of my life. Now, what I want you to do is to teach me how to change all of that."

I laughed, but actually I was a bit taken back at the time by this response. In making his request, this man was being perfectly serious, and although I smiled, privately I felt rather nervous. I must say that I was, on the one hand, flattered; first, that he thought I was right and, second, that he seemed to think that if I understood the problem, I must also have the answer. On the other hand, what he wanted seemed like an awfully tall order. While I did feel that I understood part of the problem that people face in their sexual relationships, I was not at all sure that I had the solution to these problems at hand. I did not have a perfect sexual relationship and I didn't know anyone who did. I did have some ideas, though, and my friend had others, and together we devised some exercises that we hoped might at least point the way towards change. What appears in this and the next two chapters are refinements of those ideas. Hopefully, they will point the way for you, too, and start you on the road toward getting more out of your sexual relationships.

The first ingredient necessary for change is most essential, and there is no therapist, book, or exercise that can give it to you. It is, simply, the desire to change. Without some basic motivation on your part, no amount of talk or reading will make a bit of difference. Changing is not easy, and usually people have mixed feelings about it. Partly this is because you can never be sure ahead of time that you're going to like all of the changes you make once you make them, or what's in store for you later on, after you change. Although the man in the adult education class seemed to have made up his mind, it is not always so simple as that for a lot of people. Trying to decide whether to stay the same, or to take a chance and change, can raise a lot of anxiety. However, in the long run, you must make a choice for yourself, and then live with it as best you can.

Aside from the worries that changing can create, the process of change is also difficult because it is not, generally speaking, comfortable. At least in the beginning, change feels uncomfortable, forced, or artificial. This is true for all sorts of changes, whether they involve sex, learning to be more assertive, changing the way you look or dress, or whatever. First steps are always awkward. They can make you feel as though you are being false or out of character, and at times they can be embarrassing. You must get past this stage if you are going to be able to make the changes you want to make. This means that you will need to push yourself to try things that seem uncomfortable or even silly at first. If you can stick with it, this stage will pass. Then, as changes begin to take hold, you may even get to the point of enjoying the process of change and discover how exciting it can really be to do something for yourself.

If you are in a relationship, change is something that concerns two people, not just one. Even if you decide that you want to change yourself, without asking your partner to change, you must realize that any changes in you will in turn affect your partner and your relationship. Moreover, some changes cannot be made alone. You cannot, for instance, change a sexual relationship by changing only *one* script. If you, as a man, would like to give up some of the responsibility and control during your sexual encounters, your partner must be willing to accept some additional responsibility and to be in control some of the time. Otherwise, nothing will happen (except that you both may end up lying back and waiting for the other one to make a move).

Change is more likely to succeed if both partners want it. If both you and your lover feel that you each stand to benefit from change, for example, by liberating yourselves from your sexual scripts, you will be more likely to succeed as a couple than you would by yourself. Your cooperative efforts, plus the chance to share your feelings with one another, will be a great help in getting through the initial awkward stages, and the excitement you can experience together later on may bring you closer. To stretch a cliché, it takes two to learn to tango, so it would be wise to try to make a joint decision about pursuing changes in your sexual relationship.

SEXUAL SCRIPTS VERSUS SEXUAL SCHEMAS

The sexual scripts that men and women have been encouraged to follow in their sexual encounters can be thought of as one *pattern* for lovemaking. As discussed earlier, there is nothing wrong with this pattern in itself, but problems can develop when it is the *only* pattern people use. In that case the limitations of these sexual scripts take their toll on men and women alike, leading to disappointment, boredom, and unhappiness, and setting the stage for sexual dysfunctions.

It would seem, therefore, that one of the keys to sexual fulfillment is for couples to be able to break free from limiting themselves to a single pattern of lovemaking. Aside from a basic desire on both parts to do this, several other factors seem important. Among these are a willingness to experiment and a concentrated effort to improve communication with one another in bed. These things will prepare you, as a couple, to begin developing patterns of lovemaking in addition to the one defined by the sexual scripts. These skills will also enable you as individuals to get more out of your sexual relationship. Several of the exercises in this chapter are designed to help you accomplish these things.

Besides working together with your partner on changing your sexual relationship, sexual fulfillment demands that men reassess their ideas about their own sexuality and that they begin to explore their sexuality in new ways. We need to challenge the notion that men are sexually insensitive—ready and able to perform anytime, anyplace, with any willing partner. To get more satisfaction out of sex, men need to move in the opposite direction: to discover more about their sexual sensitivities and to act on that knowledge. One place to begin is the area of sexual interest, where we can learn something about what sorts of things seem to turn us on and off sexually. Another good starting point is our bodies, which most men do not really know very well, at least not from a sexual standpoint. These two goals—discovering more about the basis of your sexual desire and the erotic potential of your own body—are the focus of this chapter.

All men are not alike sexually. This may seem like a simple enough statement, but in fact it is a revolutionary idea. Traditionally, men (and women as well) have been thought to be pretty much identical sexually: men are all turned on by the same sort of thing and have bodies that respond equally to the same sorts of stimulation. For example, it has been thought that most men are turned on by the same few "types" of women. And these types, which are really very similar to one another in many ways, are therefore thrown at us continually in books, movies, television, and advertising. Similarly, it has been assumed that all men equally enjoy being touched in certain ways in certain places on their bodies.

Simple observation of couples reveals that, to the contrary, different men are in fact attracted to different sorts of women (as are women to different sorts of men). Also, talking in depth to men reveals that they do not all like to be touched in the same ways, and that the more a man discovers about his body, the more different and individual his preferences become from those of other men. Despite these facts, however, the stereotypes about male sexuality persist. People continue to think that men are sexually simple: easily aroused, insensitive to circumstances, more concerned with physical pleasure than love, and so on. Such ideas are reflections of the broader male sex role, which was touched on in chapter 1 and which concerns the kinds of traits we have traditionally tried to develop in men. It is true that, in some measure, trying to act like a "proper man" requires you to suppress certain feelings. Men are competitive with one another, and this requires them to try, starting from early age, to overcome feelings such as fear and pain. Being competitive also prevents them from getting emotionally close to one another; to be, in a word, vulnerable to one another. Because they try to overcome, minimize, or deny certain feelings, however, does not mean that men don't have them. Just as you can't judge a book by its cover, you can't judge a man solely by his outward manner. Personal experience, as well as experience in working with men, is convincing proof that men do feel emotions such as fear, pain, loneliness, weakness, shyness, and vulnerability. They also do try to control, overcome, or deny such feelings except in unusual circumstances, such as in an intimate relationship with a woman.

So, despite their image and in spite of their efforts to minimize it, men do have their "soft side." In trying to deny this part of them, they pay a price. Sexually, trying to deny your sensitivity and perform like a sexual machine is, ultimately, a losing proposition. In one way or another, sooner or later, your sensitivities will make an appearance. You may develop sexual dysfunction, or you may not. In either case, your sensitivities, if you deny them, are likely to surface in the form of feelings of disappointment, frustration, and unhappiness with your sexual relationship. Rather than deny them, then, it would better serve your interests to try to learn more about your sensitivities, which means discovering more about your unique sexuality as an individual man. This is where the idea of *sexual schemas* comes in.

It would seem a fair statement to say that, as a unique individual, the sorts of things that might turn me on sexually would be at least slightly different from the things that could turn you on. Similarly, the way in which I experience my body—the particular ways in which it gives me pleasure—would probably be at least slightly different from the things you enjoy most. I might, for example, be attracted to serious, mysterious women and like to have my ears licked, while you might be more attracted to lighthearted, athletic women and not enjoy having your ears licked so much as your nipples. In some ways we might share some preferences; in other areas our individual sexualities may differ a lot. We might both like to kiss, but I might like to have sex on the floor with the lights on, while you might prefer it in bed with the lights out. You might like anal intercourse, I might not, and so on. Taken together, all those things that make up my sexual preferences constitute *my* sexual schema; all those things that make up your preferences and that define your individual sexuality constitute *your* sexual schema. Each of us has a sexual schema that is, as a whole, unique to us.

Learning more about your individual sexual preferences—your sexual schema—is what this chapter is about. We will focus on four main areas: three have to do with the kinds of women to whom you are likely to be sexually attracted, and one concerns your own physical sensuality. In each case you will be asked to do an exercise whose aim is to help you discover more about your sexual sensitivities. Remember the ideas behind these exercises: Men are not all turned on by the same things, nor do their bodies all respond in the same way; the more you are able to fulfill your own sexual preferences in your sexual encounters, the more satisfying your sexual relationship will be. In other words, the more your particular relationship fits your own sexual schema, the more fulfilling it will be for you. This goes for your partner as well, of course. By giving more thought than you may have in the past to the sorts of things that do turn you on, and by learning more about your own body, you will be gaining knowledge that you can apply to improving the quality of your sexual relationship. Although these exercises are written for men, they may be of interest to women as well. Your partner, too, has a sexual schema, and she can also benefit from learning more about it.

DIMENSIONS OF SEXUAL INTEREST

Men are not always sexually turned on. They are not always ready for, and looking for, sex. They do not have bodies that can be turned on by just anyone, anytime, anyplace. Rather than being insensitive sexual machines, men are complex human beings who have many sensitivities. One part of them is their sexuality, and some men (and women) may in fact have a naturally stronger sex "drive" than others. However, this sex drive is not blind. A man's sexual desire is aroused when a woman meets his particular sexual preferences, that is, when she fits that part of his sexual schema that has to do with sexual interest. The more a particular woman fits his schema, the more sexually attracted a man will be to her. Conversely, the less she fits, the less intense his attraction will be.

There are, of course, many different qualities in a woman that might attract a man. There are, in fact, so many different factors that can play a part in sexual desire that there would not be room enough in any book to discuss them all. But let us focus on three factors that are related to sexual attraction and that seem to be particularly important. These factors are physical appearance, character, and the nature of your relationship. Together, individual preferences in these three areas form the core of that part of a person's sexual schema that has to do with feeling sexual desire. Exploring these parts of your sexual schema is the purpose of the following exercises.

Exercise 2.1: Physical Attributes and Sexual Interest

Our traditional ideas about male sexuality, which are reflected in popular books, magazines, films, television, fashion, and so on, suggest that men pretty much like the same things. For example, they are supposed to like (these days) long hair, thin ankles, and high cheekbones. Although a man may in part be turned on by physical attributes such as these, his true tastes and preferences will always remain somewhat unique and might not always agree with the stereotypes in books, films, and other media.

It may not be easy to discover one's true personal preferences, since a man's ideas about what he "really" likes will always be colored by the things he learned as an adolescent. At the same time that boys learn their sexual scripts, they develop ideas about what is (and is not) physically attractive. Adolescent boys spend a lot of time talking about female physical appearance. In the process, they tend to reach a consensus about what is and what is not attractive. As guides, they use pictures of "beautiful" women from magazines, movies, and television which are, of course, all stereotypes, and so their individual preferences tend to get lost. Despite this tendency, it is possible for a man to discover something about his individual sexual preferences if he is willing to give it some thought.

Men not only differ in their preferences—*what* they like—but also in terms of *how important* a woman's different physical attributes are to their sexual interest. Again, there are some stereotypes that would lead us to believe that all men value certain physical attributes equally. For example, a long-held stereotype suggests that legs and breasts are very important. In fact, these things are not equally important to all men. Individual differences in the importance that any one man places on a woman's various physical attributes are usually revealed by what he will notice first, second, third, and so on about a particular woman. Usually, men will check out first what is for them the most important thing, then second, the next most important thing, and so on. Whether they end up feeling sexually attracted then depends on just how important each thing they see is to them (that is, whether it is a little important or very important), and, of course, whether a particular woman's appearance fits their preference. Some men may find breasts and legs extremely important, and if these things on a particular woman are not "right" for them, they will not feel sexually attracted to that woman no matter how she looks otherwise. Other men seem to weigh their preferences more evenly. They may be able to focus on those things that "fit" their schema and ignore those things that don't and, therefore, feel turned on to many women.

Try to give some thought now not only to what you find attractive and unattractive in women, but also to how important each of your preferences is to you. You may find this exercise difficult at first. It will be especially difficult if you have not thought much about this sort of thing before. Also, your thinking will probably be clouded by the stereotypes you learned years ago—the ideas you got as an adolescent about what you should find attractive. In doing this exercise, however, give thought to everything you write down to try to get in touch with what you actually like, rather than what you think you should like.

Doing this exercise correctly takes time and undivided attention, and it probably should be done in private. It may take you an hour or longer to complete it thoroughly, and you may not be able to finish it in one sitting. Give yourself this time. Also, try to be as honest with yourself as possible. Don't worry if other men, or anyone else for that matter, would agree or disagree with your personal tastes. The Physical Attributes Schema Chart has been designed as an aid to you in your work. Go through it carefully and fill it out according to the guides below.

> *Imagine for a moment several women you know (or have known) whose physical appearances you find sexually attractive, as well as several whose physical appearances do not particularly attract you. If you can, picture these women in your mind. Take about fifteen minutes to do this. Remember to think about both attractive and unattractive women on a physical level only.*
>
> *Try to identify* differences *in the physical appearances of the women you are sexually interested in as compared to those you are not. Look for things that are attractive (seem to turn you on), as well as things that are unattractive (seem to turn you off). On the chart, line 1, write a description of the first difference you can think of. If the difference is something that is a turn-on—an attractive quality—write the description in the Attractive column; if it is a physical attribute that turns you off, write the description in the Unattractive column. For example, if you believe that one of the things common to many of the women to whom you are attracted is that they are thin, write that in the Attractive column as physical attribute 1; if you think of thick ankles as one physical attribute that turns you off, write that as attribute 2 under Unattractive, and so on. In this way you can build your personal list of physical attributes, some turn-ons and others turn-offs. Hopefully, you will be able to list a total of at least ten such personal preferences.*

Some people have an easier time being able to picture things in their minds than others. If you happen to be a person who can't do this very well, it might be a good idea to spend some time *tactfully* looking at some real women before doing this exercise. As you do so, notice things that you seem to find both attractive and unattractive.

PHYSICAL ATTRIBUTES SCHEMA CHART

	Attractive	*Unattractive*	*Importance*
1			1 2
2			1 2
3			1 2
4			1 2
5			1 2
6			1 2
7			1 2
8			1 2
9			1 2
10			1 2

Your physical attributes schema is now half complete. You have built a list of descriptions of physical attributes that partly determine whether you will be sexually attracted to, or not attracted to, a particular woman. There is also an additional factor that enters into this schema, and that is how *important* each preference listed is to you personally.

For some men, it is very important that a woman's physical appearance conforms to their preferences in every way. If even one thing is "wrong," these men are not sexually attracted. Usually, the things that are turn-offs are more critical than the things that are turn-ons. If a woman happens to have a physical attribute that turns men off, they will not be sexually interested in her. Other men have schemas that are more flexible. They may have preferences about the way a woman looks, both positive and negative, but it is not so important that a woman fit all of these preferences. More than that, if a woman's body happens to include some attribute that is a turn-off for them, they can still be attracted to her *if* she fits their preferences in some other ways. These men, in short, need to have at least some of their positive preferences for physical attributes fulfilled in order to feel sexual desire for a woman, but they are not thrown off by something that does not "fit." Such men can usually focus their attention on the attributes that do fit their schema and ignore those that don't. Of course, the more their preferences are met, the more strongly attracted they will be.

There also may be a few men for whom a woman's physical appearance does not play a role in determining their sexual desire. These men (probably extremely few) would be able to feel sexually attracted to a woman whose physical appearance did not fit their preferences in any way. In a sense, these men have no preferences. Their physical attributes charts should actually be blank, or else filled in with just anything, which they know does not really matter to them at all.

To finish your personal physical attributes schema, go through the chart again, beginning with physical attribute 1, and assign each attribute listed an *importance rating*—either a 1 or a 2—using the system below.

Importance Rating	Meaning
1	*Critical.* If a woman's appearance is wrong for you in this particular area, you will not be sexually attracted to her no matter what she is like otherwise.
2	*Important But Not Critical.* If a woman's appearance is wrong for you in this particular area, you can feel sexually attracted to her if her appearance is right in other ways.

Your description of your personal preferences in physical appearances is now complete. This particular schema may change in the future, but the way it appears in the chart is the way it is for you now. Take some time to look through it. The guidelines that follow are intended to give you some idea about possible implications of your preferences for your own sex life.

The more times you circle 1 in the chart, the more *demanding* your physical attributes schema is. In other words, the more 1's you circle, the more "fussy" you are. The most extreme case would be a man who circles all 1's. By doing this, he is saying that in order for him to feel sexually attracted to a woman, her physical appearance has to fit each and every one of his preferences; if even one thing is not right about her appearance, he will not feel sexual desire. The problem facing such men is finding women whose physical appearances fit that particular schema in such detail—who have all of the qualities they like and none of the qualities they don't like. Although such men are rare, I have spoken with some who seemed to be in this category, or close to it, and they give the impression that it is a real bind for them. Frequently, they are unable to find even one woman who is right for them in every way. Or, if they do find such a woman and feel sexually attracted to her, a problem develops later on when her body, like theirs, begins to change. Unless their schema changes, too, their once-perfect partner sooner or later becomes imperfect, and these men lose their sexual interest.

Circling even a single 1 on your chart means, of course, that you have at least one personal preference that just has to be met in order for you to feel sexual desire for a woman. It may be something positive (a physical attribute that a woman must possess in order for you to feel turned on), or it may be something negative (something that always turns you off). Any schema that has at least one such critical element may be called a *rigid* schema. There are more men with schemas in this category than the first one. It may be something as simple as the thickness of an ankle, the curve of a calf, the size of the breasts, or the length of the hair, but whatever it is, it has to be right or the man is not sexually interested. It may be difficult for a man to admit that this one thing (which is almost always the very first thing he looks at) is so important to him, but the truth is that it is. Usually, such men do not have too much trouble finding women who pass the critical test, and so their physical attributes schema does not limit or handicap them as it does for a man who has an extremely demanding one.

Most men seem to have physical attributes schemas of the following sort: for them to feel sexual desire for a woman, her physical appearance has to fit at least some of their preferences; the more preferences she fits, the more attracted they will be. She may have some qualities that are negatives for them, but so long as the positives outweigh the negatives, they can feel attracted. These men do not have any critical preferences—preferences that absolutely have to be met. Such schemas can be called *flexible*.

If you have not circled any 1's in your chart and have circled only 2's, you have a flexible physical attributes schema. So long as a woman does fit more of your positive than negative preferences, chances are that she will arouse some sexual interest. Naturally, the more positives she has, and the fewer negatives, the more attracted you will be.

Depending upon the physical attributes, men with flexible schemas may be able to ignore or downplay those attributes in a woman that do not fit their particular preferences. At the same time, they can concentrate attention on those qualities that do fit their preferences. This may be a technique for men who have rigid schemas to use, in order to become more flexible.

Earlier we mentioned the possibility that sexual interest schemas may change over time. It may have already occurred to you that your physical attributes schema as it is today differs from what it once was. This may not be true for all men; for some, the schema stays pretty much the same. What might be responsible for change in some and not in others is difficult to say. It is true that, for many of us, our values change as we age.

And it makes sense that changing values can affect our sexuality. Physical appearances as a whole may become less important as we get older, and/or one may become more flexible. It may be possible, too, for men to alter their sexual schemas on purpose if they want to. This could be in your interest, especially if you are a man who has one or more critical conditions as part of your schema.

The best approach to attempting any change (to go from rigid to flexible) is to see if you can find some things that do appeal to you in the way a woman looks, and then focus your attention on those. You may be able to find any number of things about a woman that are appealing. There may, of course, be things about her appearance that do not appeal to you, or which turn you off. You may find that it is possible for you to focus on the things that contribute to your sexual interest, while ignoring those things that don't. If this happens, and your interest is aroused but wanes, it may be that your attention has drifted back to something that is a negative for you. In that case, try shifting to the positive. You may need to work on this technique for some time before it will work, and for some men it may not work at all, but it is worthwhile trying.

It may also be possible for a woman to change something about her physical appearance to fit a particular man's preferences more closely. If it is something that turns her partner off, yet seems changeable, a woman might want to consider this option. If there is something about your partner that you realize is turning you off sexually, and if shifting your attention to the positive does not seem to work, it may be helpful to discuss the problem. Before you do this, however, give it some serious thought. Consider how you would feel if the roles were reversed—if your partner told you that something in your looks turned her off. Nobody likes to be told that there is something unappealing about them, so you would be wise to say so in a way that you might want to be told.

If the physical attribute that is turning you off is one that you don't think your partner can change, or if your desires would require a drastic change, your dilemma is obviously worse than if it is something that could be changed. In that case, you may want to make a real effort at focusing on other things before you consider confronting your partner with your feelings.

Some readers may object to the notion of a physical attributes schema and to this exercise. It may seem to be encouraging men to "objectify" women. This is not the intention. The assumption that underlies this exercise is, simply, that men do have personal preferences and that the ways in which a woman's appearance does or does not fit those preferences partly determine male sexual desire. Since these schemas do exist, there seems little to be gained in pretending otherwise. Moreover, women as well as men have such schemas.

The physical attributes schema described in this exercise, however, is only one factor, as we will see, that goes into determining whether you will be sexually interested in a particular woman. Although it may be important, it is rarely the only factor that influences your sexual interest. The set of personal preferences you worked out here is part of your individual sexuality. They may be similar in ways to those of other men, but your preferences taken together are probably unique and set you apart from others. Hopefully, at this point, you can begin thinking of yourself in these terms (as a unique individual rather than a carbon copy). In addition, while doing this first exercise, you may begin to appreciate your sexual sensitivity. Your physical attributes schema is evidence of this sensitivity. It suggests that your sexual desire does not spring solely from some uncontrollable instinct, but that it is in large measure influenced by circumstances, in this case a woman's physical appearance.

Exercise 2.2: Character and Sexual Interest

A second factor that influences sexual desire has to do with the sorts of personal qualities an individual possesses. The term *character* refers to all personal qualities, such as trustworthiness, aggressiveness, modesty, and so on, that typify a person's behavior and life-style. The idea of a *character schema* is similar to the idea of a physical attributes schema. In one case, we are talking about a set of physical attributes you find attractive; in the other case, it is a set of personal qualities you find attractive.

As we know, men differ in how important physical appearance is to their sexual interest. In going through Exercise 2.1, you may have discovered that the way a woman looks plays an important role in determining whether you will be drawn to her, or you may have discovered that it plays a minor role in determining your sexual interest. And even when it turns out to be important, physical appearance is seldom, if ever, the only thing that determines sexual interest. A second factor that typically enters the picture is character. If it pleases you, a woman's character will enhance your attraction to her, and if it does not, your sexual interest will be reduced.

Focus your attention now on trying to identify some of the personal qualities a woman may have that would lead you to feel sexually attracted or not attracted to her. Again, there is a chart to aid you.

> *You can begin to build a description of your character schema by taking fifteen minutes or so to think about women, in this case, all of whom you think are physically attractive, but only some of whom you are sexually interested in. In other words, think of some women you find physically attractive, but who do not interest you sexually, as well as some in whom you are sexually interested.*
>
> *It is likely that your different reactions to these women (attraction versus nonattraction) is in part due to differences in their personal qualities or character. Think about this. Try to identify some differences between the women you are sexually interested in and those you are not. Concentrate, of course, not on differences in physical appearance, but on differences in personal qualities, character, or life-style.*

When you think you have identified one such difference, write a description of it in the Character Schema Chart, in the appropriate column (Attractive or Unattractive). Begin with personal quality 1 and work your way down, filling in as many spaces as you can. For example, if you feel that one of the differences in character between women in whom you are sexually interested versus those you are not is that the ones you are attracted to are independent and working, write that down under Attractive. Next, if you conclude that the women you do not find sexually interesting seem to be shy, write that down, as personal quality 2, in the column beneath the heading Unattractive. If you then think that you are attracted to women who like to have parties and dance, write that down as 3 in the Attractive column. If you think you don't like women who tend to be serious, put that on your list as 4, in the Unattractive *column. In this way you will build a list of attractive and unattractive personal qualities similar to the attractive and unattractive physical attributes you listed as part of the last exercise.*

When you have finished your list of personal preferences, go through it again and, as in Exercise 2.1, assign each item an *importance rating* (1 or 2).

Importance Rating	Meaning
1	*Critical.* If a woman's character does not fit your preferences in this particular area, you will not be sexually interested in her no matter what she is like otherwise.
2	*Important But Not Critical.* If a woman's character is wrong for you in this particular area, you can feel sexual desire for her if her character is right in other ways.

When you have finished going through the chart a second time and have assigned importance ratings to all those personal qualities that seem to matter to your sexual interest, your character schema is finished. The following guides will aid you in appreciating the importance of this schema for your own sexuality.

First, go through your chart and see how many 1's you circled. As in Exercise 2.1, the more 1's your schema contains, the more *demanding* it is. Men who circle many 1's are saying that, in order for them to feel sexually attracted to a woman, her personality must fit their preferences in all of these ways. If her character does not include some critical quality they find attractive, or if it does include one they find unattractive, these men will not feel sexually interested.

CHARACTER SCHEMA CHART

	Attractive	Unattractive	Importance
1			1 2
2			1 2
3			1 2
4			1 2
5			1 2
6			1 2
7			1 2
8			1 2
9			1 2
10			1 2

Men who have extremely demanding character schemas—a large number of critical preferences—are rare. They are like the men who have very demanding physical attributes schemas in that it is usually very difficult for them to find a woman whose personality fits such a large number of critical preferences. Also, if they do find such a woman and feel attracted to her, there is the danger that her personality will change, as many people's do, and that at some point it will no longer fit their schema. The situation is, of course, even worse if the man also happens to have a highly demanding physical attributes schema. It may be next to impossible for any one woman to meet so many critical preferences in both physical appearance and character.

Somewhat more common are men for whom one or two personal qualities are critical. If you have circled even a single 1 on your chart, you fall into this category. Your character schema is *rigid;* you are saying that a woman's personality absolutely must fit your preferences in this one way. If it is a quality you are attracted to, but she doesn't have it, you are not likely to be interested in her; if it is something you don't like and she has it, you will feel turned off. Because your character schema is not as demanding as that of someone who has many critical preferences, however, the chances of finding women who do meet your critical needs are greater. But you are still limited to some extent by your critical need.

Men who have one or two critical preferences in both their physical attributes and character schemas are not uncommon. They are usually able to find women, although perhaps not a lot of them, whose physical appearance and personality both pass the critical tests. Again, they are limited in the number of women they might potentially be sexually attracted to because of their critical needs, but their situation is usually far from impossible. However, potential problems do seem to arise for these men when they encounter a woman who passes the critical test in one schema but not the other, or who changes over time so that she no longer passes the critical test in one area or the other.

The majority of men fall into a third category. They have a set of preferences, at least *some* of which need to be met in order for them to be sexually interested in a woman, but they have no critical preferences. In short, their character schemas are *flexible*. If you have circled a series of 2's, but have circled no 1's on your chart, your own schema falls into this category. Assuming that a woman's personality fits some of your important positive preferences, and assuming that these outweigh any negatives in her character, you will feel sexually interested in her. One result of this flexibility is that you can feel sexually attracted to a relatively large number of women. Naturally, the more positives and the fewer negatives a woman has, the stronger will be your attraction to her.

So far we have discussed two components of sexual interest: the physical attributes schema and the character schema. Men with flexible schemas in both areas (no critical elements in either one) have the potential to be attracted to a large number of women. They are in the opposite position of men whose physical attributes and character schemas are both rigid and demanding. In between are men who have one or two critical needs in both schemas, or who are flexible in one but rigid in the other. Where in this scheme of things do you seem to fit?

Men for whom personality traits are truly not important—who can be sexually attracted to a woman no matter what kinds of personal qualities she has—are extremely rare, but they may exist. Their charts should really be blank, since for them it makes no difference what a woman's character is like. Instead, other factors—for instance, the physical attributes schema—undoubtedly exert a much more powerful influence on their sexual interest. Unless you fall into this rare group, however, your personal preferences in the area of personality contribute to your overall sexual interest.

Through this exercise, you hopefully have been able to discover something about this particular schema as it is for you now. For some men, these preferences will remain pretty much the same throughout their lives, and if theirs happens to be a demanding and/or rigid schema, it is likely to be a permanent handicap. In other men, preferences change over time. What men like in a woman's character at age twenty-five is not always what they like in a woman at age thirty-five or older. This is probably a natural part of maturing and, in this case, the change in the schema follows personal growth in a natural way. Aside from this sort of natural change, it may be possible for men to alter their character schemas through purposeful effort. If their schemas are demanding or rigid, making them either less demanding or flexible may be a useful goal. The technique to do this is the same used to make changes in a physical attributes schema—try to focus on those personal qualities that please you and stimulate your sexual interest, while turning your attention away from those that detract from your desire. When you find your attention drifting back to a turn-off, shift to a positive. If you work at it consistently, you may discover that it is possible for you to change any 1's you originally had circled into 2's. This would place you in a position where it could be possible for you to feel sexually attracted to more women and/or to maintain your interest in one woman over time as her character changes.

Personal attraction and *sexual* attraction do not always coincide, and when this happens it may lead people toward unintegrated or split life-styles. To see if this might be true for you, go through your chart again and look at those traits you described as being sexually attractive. Try to imagine a woman who possesses a great number of these qualities. If you can, picture such a woman in your mind. Think of a woman you might know, or once knew, who fits this image. Then take some time mentally to compare those women you are (or have been) sexually involved with to your image of women who are sexually exciting to you. How well do the personalities of those women fit your schema of what is sexually appealing? Hopefully, the fit will be reasonably good. However, if a woman with whom you have an intimate relationship has a personality that does not fit your schema very well, you may have a conflict. If you are sexually attracted to this woman, your situation may be that what you think you are attracted to (what is written in your chart) is not actually what you are attracted to. In that case, you may want to reevaluate your preferences in this area.

On the other hand, if you have felt that you are not attracted, or have experienced a loss of attraction, one reason may have to do with the notion of character and how it affects sexual desire. Perhaps your partner's personality has attracted you to her in some ways (for example, as a wife), but not in a sexual way. Or, you may have been sexually attracted by her personality at one time, but you have changed your preferences since then. Finally, it is possible that your partner has changed—that she is different now from the way she once was, and some of these changes may have affected your sexual interest in her. Obviously, this represents a serious problem for your relationship, and the solution may not be an easy one. It may be possible for your partner to change, but this may not be something she wants to do (would you?).

An alternative is for you to reassess your feelings about her personality. You might, for instance, be able to discover additional qualities that you like about her. Assuming that there are at least some qualities about your partner that do appeal to you, you may be able to use the focusing technique described earlier to increase your sexual interest. This is a process that involves learning to concentrate on the things that you like, at least when you want to feel sexually turned on, while paying less attention to those things you feel less positive about. It may also be useful for the two of you to talk about your feelings at this point, perhaps with the aid of a marriage counselor.

Exercise 2.3: Relationships and Sexual Interest

To this point we have considered two factors that very likely influence sexual desire—physical appearance and personal qualities. In this exercise we will focus on yet a third factor, which concerns the *kind of relationship* you may find sexually appealing. The idea is that the terms of the relationship you have, or might have, with a woman influence your sexual desire within that relationship.

The kinds of relationships that can exist between men and women can vary, among other ways, in terms of *sexual exclusivity*. At one extreme is the most sexually exclusive form of relationship—*monogamy*. It may or may not involve a formal marriage contract, but in either case, two people in a monogamous relationship agree to have no other sexual partners but each other. Having sex with someone outside of the relationship is prohibited by mutual agreement. This, then, is *one* way in which the relationship is special, and each partner is special to the other. For some (perhaps many) couples, their sexual exclusivity is not only one, but the *only* way in which they are special to each other. Or, if it is not the only way in which they are special, it forms the cornerstone of their relationship—the most important way in which they are special to each other. When this happens, sexual infidelity on one of their parts often creates a severe crisis in the relationship. In contrast, if each partner is special to the other in additional ways (that is, not only because they are an exclusive sexual partner), so that the relationship is special in many ways, the crisis resulting from a flirtation or affair is likely to be much less severe. Similarly, if other ways in which the relationship is special are valued as highly as is sexual exclusivity, the chances of it surviving a crisis are much greater. Unfortunately, we all too often seem to use monogamy (sexual exclusivity) as either the sole basis, or else the cornerstone, of our relationships.

People who are not attracted to monogamy may feel it is limiting and may find that the idea of being sexually faithful to one and only one person has a negative effect on their sexual interest in that person. Traditionally, monogamy has been encouraged, to say the least, but it is increasingly becoming only one alternative a couple may choose. It is certainly not the only basis on which two people can form a committed relationship; nor is it the only way in which two people can be special to one another. There may, in fact, be ways that are much more important than that.

At the opposite extreme to monogamy are relationships in which there is no sexual exclusivity, the best example of which is probably *prostitution*. The terms of the relationship here are that a fee, paid by the man to the woman, is considered a fair exchange for his use of her body and the pleasure he gets from it. Once the fee is paid and he reaches orgasm (or gets whatever else he paid for), the transaction is complete. Both partners are then totally free to go their separate ways, at least sexually. Any sense of specialness that may (and sometimes does) develop within such a relationship obviously does not have sexual exclusivity as its cornerstone.

Between the two extremes of monogamy and prostitution are relationships that involve varying degrees of commitment and sexual exclusivity. Sometimes the commitment, as mentioned earlier, is related to the terms of the sexual relationship, but it does not have to be. In an *open marriage,* for example, there is one "primary" partner plus any number of "secondary" partners (one person whom you feel committed to and want to stay with forever, plus a series of lovers whom you may or may not feel committed to, but who are, in either case, not as important to you as the primary partner). As in monogamy, people living in an open marriage may have a formal (legal) commitment, or their commitment may be only personal. Their sense of specialness, again, is not founded on being each other's sole sexual partner, but must be rooted instead in other aspects of the relationship.

Moving from open marriage in the direction of decreasing sexual exclusivity, there are relationships with *lovers:* people whom you care about and may feel emotionally involved with, (even committed to) but to whom you do not feel bound to be sexually faithful. The "affair" may last for a long time, but neither partner is special to the other in the same sense as is true in either open or monogamous marriages. Needless to say, any sense of specialness about a relationship with a lover is not based on having each other as sole sexual partners.

Less commitment to the relationship is involved in so-called *recreational sex.* The motive for a sexual encounter or relationship here is mutual pleasure, period. There is an expectation that both partners will derive some pleasure from having a sexual encounter, and each accepts this goal of mutual enjoyment as partly his or her responsibility. Beyond this, recreational sex implies neither commitment not sexual exclusivity. After the sexual encounter, both partners are free to go their separate ways. There can still be an intense emotional investment made, even when sex is undertaken in a recreational way, although this investment is obviously a brief one.

For people to feel as much sexual desire for a partner as they might, they need to feel right about the relationship. If the terms on which a sexual relationship or encounter is based feel "wrong" to you, this will detract from any sexual interest you might experience.

How attractive do you personally find each of the above types of relationships? For you to appreciate fully your own *relationship schema,* go through the list below and, in the blanks provided, assign each of the alternative relationship types an *attraction rating,* from 1 to 3, using the following system.

Attraction Rating	Meaning
1	*Critical.* This is the only kind of relationship that appeals to you.
2	*Attractive But Not Critical.* This kind of relationship has a definite appeal to you, but you are attracted to other sorts of relationships as well.
3	*Unattractive.* This particular variety of relationship definitely does not appeal to you.

Sexual Relationship List

Monogamy _____
Open Marriage _____
Lovers _____
Recreational Sex _____
Prostitution _____

When you have finished going through the list and assigning attraction ratings, take some time to look it over. The following guidelines are intended as an aid in understanding the implications of these ratings for you.

Men who have assigned only an attraction rating of 1, giving all other relationship types ratings of 3, have what amounts to the simplest or least complicated relationship schema. They are strongly drawn to one and only one type of relationship, and they have no conflict within themselves, at least in terms of what they want. In the context of the sort of relationship they prefer, they will experience sexual desire, but in other relational contexts they will not. If it is monogamy that attracts them, such men will not find the possibility of recreational sex to be a turn-on. Similarly, if they are drawn to recreational sex, they will not tend to feel sexual desire for a woman who would prefer a monogamous relationship.

Men who have not assigned any relationship type a rating of 1, but have given out one or more 2's, may or may not experience conflict, depending on which relationships get which ratings. Obviously, if you gave a positive rating (2) to both monogamy and *any* other type of relationship, you have a conflict. Of all the relationships listed above, only monogamy is inconsistent with wanting any of the others. There is little or no conflict involved when you are attracted both to lovers and recreational sex, or open marriage and lovers. The situation is quite different, however, when a person feels drawn both to monogamy and anything else. One way to resolve such a conflict is to see if one type of relationship appeals to you more than the other, and then to pursue this one, letting the other one go. Although this is easy to say, it is anything but easy to do, and it often takes people years to resolve such a conflict within themselves. During this time their sexual relationship, if they are monogamous, may suffer. For people who prefer monogamy, sexual interest will be affected by the status or quality of their "marriage" at any given time. If they are feeling good about the relationship, their sexual desire will be strong and their sexual relationship will be more or less fulfilling. It will bring them closer, and it will reaffirm and be a reflection of their love and emotional investment in each other. If, however, one partner is not feeling good about the relationship, his or her sexual interest is likely to suffer as a consequence. Although it is certainly difficult, their best alternative at such times is to realize what is happening to them and try to resolve whatever it is that is making them feel bad.

Our culture has in the past—and to a good degree still does—advocate monogamy as the best type of relationship between a man and a woman. For those people who are not personally attracted to it, however, monogamy can have negative effects on their sexuality. Today, there are more alternatives available to such persons than there used to be. If you feel that you are one such individual, your situation may or may not be problematic, depending on whether you are attempting to be monogamous. If you are, then unless you become more attracted to the idea of sexual exclusivity, the terms of your relationship will detract from your sexual desire. If you are not currently in an exclusive relationship, you would do best to consider your preferences in this area before you make any such commitment.

One alternative available to persons who feel limited by monogamy, and whose sexual desire suffers as a result, is to move from it toward an open marriage. This is not an easy alternative to pursue, partly because it is, in a sense, more risky than conventional monogamy. The risk is, of course, that one or both partners may leave one "primary" partner for another. Open marriage seems more complex than traditional monogamy, and something that at the very least demands a great deal of compromise, plus an ability to deal with feelings of jealousy and insecurity; this is because, as mentioned earlier, we have made sex into such an important component of our relationships. To be successful, an open marriage must be open in other ways besides sex—communication, for example. Finally, couples who choose an open marriage must be able to base their feelings of specialness (to each other) on things other than sexual exclusivity. For all of these reasons, open marriages often do not work out in the long run; that is, the partners separate. That is probably not because open marriage is a bad idea, period. Rather, open marriages often seem to fail because they are doomed from the beginning—a last-ditch effort to save a dying marriage, or because one or both partners were not able to find anything to substitute for sexual exclusivity as a way of making the relationship special. Therefore, persons who are considering open marriage should first think about whether they may want to open the marriage as a way of saving it. If so, they should be aware that this approach often backfires. If you are unhappy in your marriage, you would probably do well to consider marriage counseling. This can lead to one of three solutions: you may decide in favor of continuing a monogamous relationship, you may move toward an open marriage, or you may separate.

A second piece of advice to couples (in this case, those who are considering open marriage as well as those who are not) is to reassess your relationship right now, from the point of view of specialness. The following exercise may be helpful in this regard.

Exercise 2.4: Specialness and Sexual Interest
One thing that has resulted from my work with couples is an impression about the role that feelings of specialness play in bonding a couple together and in the couple's sexual interest.

> Bob and Carol were married for about ten years. Neither had what you could call a normal upbringing, in the sense that neither had a family whom, they felt, cared about them. As adolescents and young adults, both had been very sexually active, but neither had experienced much emotional involvement in these early relationships. They came to therapy because, for about three years, Bob's interest in sex had been steadily dropping off to the point where the couple now rarely had any sexual, or even affectionate contact with each other. This situation was in sharp contrast to the years before, when sex and affection had been frequent and satisfying for both of them.
>
> When I interviewed them, both partners dated the onset of the problem to the time, three years earlier, when Bob had lost his

job under uncomfortable circumstances in which (for about six months) he also faced possible legal action. Although it did not occur to me to explore this area in depth at first, after a few sessions I decided to explore the history of this relationship from the perspective of specialness. Specifically, I asked Bob to explain to me what initially attracted him to Carol and what, in his opinion, had kept them together. In other words, I wanted him to tell me how their relationship, both initially and later on, was special for him.

Bob's first response was to say that he was initially attracted to Carol mainly because of her looks, that is, it was a physical attraction. Although this seemed reasonable enough, I also felt that there must have been some additional qualities in Carol and in their relationship that made him begin to feel serious about it after awhile. Did he really believe, I asked, that his desire to pursue and marry Carol was based purely on her looks? It took some time, but Bob eventually came up with two ideas. The first was that he had felt, from the beginning, that he could help to save Carol from what he saw as a self-destructive life-style (drugs) and could offer her something better. Second, he was aware that Carol admired him and that she was totally behind him in anything he wanted to do.

As you might guess, my next questions to the couple concerned what impact Bob's job trouble had on the feeling that he could take care of Carol and be respected by her. Needless to say, both acknowledged that the experience had shaken them considerably. Bob had felt Carol withdraw some of her unqualified support from him and he worried that he would not be able to pick up the pieces and start again. In many ways (and for reasons that are not important here) they had never really resolved that crisis, and Bob had withdrawn slowly but steadily ever since.

The case of Bob and Carol illustrates the point that specialness is not only the basis of a bond between two people, but that it also affects their sexual relationship. A colleague and friend is fond of saying that one of the most fundamental human needs is the "need to be needed"; in short, to be special to someone else. Bob and Carol had this, at least at first. Interestingly, sexual exclusivity was not a part of this foundation, or at least it did not seem to be. Although both were sexually faithful, the other things that Bob talked about seemed to be much more important than exclusivity. It was my guess that he could have coped with his wife having an affair much better than he had been able to cope with the loss of the other aspects of specialness that resulted from his job crisis.

To assess the role of specialness in your own relationship and to see if it is founded on more things than sexual exclusivity, give some thought now to what, in your opinion, resulted in your feeling *serious* about your current partner. Try to identify what was *special* about her and your relationship. What sorts of qualities did *she* have that seemed to set her apart, in your own mind, from other women? How did she treat you that made *you* feel special to her?

> Ways in which my partner was special (different from other women) that made me feel serious about my relationship with her: _____
> _____
> _____
>
> Ways in which my partner treated me that made *me* feel special to her: _____
> _____
> _____
> _____

When you finish writing down your thoughts on what was special about your relationship in the beginning, write down your thoughts about your relationship as it is *now*.

> Ways in which my partner is special to me now: _____
> _____
> _____
> _____
> _____

Ways in which my partner treats me now that make me feel special: _____

_____

_____

_____

Now compare your two lists. If you feel ready for such a discussion, have your partner prepare two lists, exchange lists, read them, and then talk about your reactions. In your thoughts (and/or discussions) try to direct yourself to each of the following questions.

- How much was the specialness in your relationship, in the beginning, based on sexual exclusivity and how much was based on other things?
- How much is the specialness in your relationship, now, based on sexual exclusivity and how much is it based on other things?
- Are the things that were sources of feelings of specialness early in your relationship still sources for such feelings today?
- Have the number of ways in which you and your partner are special to one another increased over time, decreased, or remained the same?
- How special do you feel to your partner these days?
- How special is your partner to you right now?
- Have there been times when the foundation of your feelings of specialness was shaken by one crisis or another (as in the case of Bob and Carol)? If so, do you believe this had an effect on your sexual relationship? Have you resolved that crisis, or is it still an open wound between you?

It seems to be difficult to *create* specialness—to make someone else special to you on purpose. On the other hand, people sometimes seem to lose sight of their specialness within a relationship, in which case this exercise may be useful. If going through it has brought you in touch with feelings of specialness that had been forgotten, it has served its purpose well. Of course, it may also be painful for some, in that it may make you aware of unresolved conflicts between (or within) you, or even that you don't feel special (or regard your partner as special) today as you once might have. Some may discover that the only way they are special is in being an exclusive sexual partner. If this is true for you, you are at least in a position now to understand your situation better. If you have lost sexual interest, and if that seems now to be related in part to this idea of specialness, you may be able to work on it together, or you may decide to seek professional help, depending on how severe the problem appears and whether working on it yourselves seems to get you anywhere.

The main point of this section is, simply, that the overall quality of your relationship most definitely influences its sexual aspect. Sexual relationships are parts of whole relationships. Depending on the quality of your relationship—whether its terms fit your preferences and whether it gives you a sense of specialness—your sexual interest within it will either flourish or wither. These exercises have been designed to help you to get in touch with these issues and point you in the direction of change, if need be.

Summing up Sexual Interest

Sexual desire is a response within yourself that is determined by a variety of factors. In the preceding sections you were asked to explore each of three such factors. Each schema is a component that goes into the making of a whole—sexual desire.

Learning about some of the factors related to your own sexual interest is a first step in the process of self-discovery. Preferences, or schemas, are personal, individual things, and while some of your own preferences may be the same as, or similar to, some other men's, chances are your sexual preferences *as a set* are unique to you. Realizing that every man's sexuality is unique and discovering something about your own sexual preferences mean stepping away from the sexual stereotypes about men that were discussed in chapter 1. Trying to make your own sexual interest fit the myth that men are sexually identical means denying at least some of your individuality. At best, the popular notion about what is attractive may fit pieces of your schemas, but they are not likely to fit all, or even most, of them very well.

The second step is to get you to begin realizing that your sexuality is sensitive. Specifically, while we all—men and women alike—have sex drives, our sexual interest is heavily influenced by many factors. Whether you will be sexually interested in a given woman may be in some part a matter of instinct, but it is even more heavily determined by things we have discussed: physical appearance, character, and the quality of your relationship. Your sexuality is affected by these things, and to improve your sense of sexual fulfillment, you must begin to think of yourself in these terms.

MALE SENSUALITY

Another strong impression that has come from experience in working with men as a sex therapist and educator is that few men fully appreciate the erotic potential of their own bodies. Compared with women, men in general have only a crude awareness of their bodies from the perspective of sensual pleasure. In contrast, men usually have a better awareness than women of their bodies from an athletic perspective. These differences between the sexes, and the ways in which they know their bodies, can be related to differences in the male versus female sex roles, that is, the different traits that men and women have been encouraged to develop. Men have always been encouraged to be physically active in a way that would lead them to learn about the skills and limitations of their bodies. They have also been encouraged to develop and maintain their physical strength. Women have been encouraged to care for their bodies in a different way. Instead of developing muscles in athletic skills, they have been encouraged to maintain their softness: to be, in a word, sensual.

The sexual scripts by which couples have traditionally patterned their sexual relationships serve to increase the differences in the ways in which men and women experience their bodies. Under the arrangement that casts the woman in the passive role, with the man doing things in order to arouse her, it makes sense that she would be more likely to learn more about her body than he might about his.

Partly as a result of their sex role and partly because of their sexual script, men are not likely to develop an awareness of their sensuality. They are not likely to be very aware of their many different erogenous zones or how they like to be touched in various places. If they did know more about themselves in these ways, they would be in a position to get that much more pleasure from sexual encounters.

A third factor that keeps men from developing their sensual awareness is also related to sexual scripts, and this has to do with the fact that men have been encouraged to be "genitally focused," concerned mainly with the pleasure they can derive from their penises and from intercourse. Women often complain that men are too anxious to have intercourse, that they don't engage in enough foreplay, and that they want to end a sexual encounter just as soon as they have had their orgasm. Although this frequently seems to be the case, it is important to keep in mind that men are not *naturally* this way. Rather, their behavior in bed largely reflects the way in which they have been encouraged to regard their bodies and the fact that intercourse has been set up as a goal—and therefore an end-all—for them.

The sexual situation that faces men is something like this: Men are raised to be the one who must take the sexual initiative in a relationship. The man comes to regard a sexual encounter as a performance, or test, as much as a pleasant experience or a chance for intimate emotional contact. When viewed in this way, a sexual encounter is like a game in which intercourse is first prize. It is little wonder, then, that other sexual activities should be less attractive to men. At the same time, men are placed in the role of getting turned on not so much by having things done to them as by doing things to their partners' bodies. Of course, a man will be kissed and his genitals may get some fondling, but it is rare for a man to get as much in the way of touching as he gives. Then, too, he rarely has an opportunity to lie back and be made love to, since he feels responsible for the sexual performance and feels the need to take the initiative.

With these considerations in mind, complaints about men's inadequacies as lovers take on a different light. It may be true that, in one sense, men have been in control in the sexual situation (because they are the ones who are given the role of initiator), but this control is far from absolute. To a large extent, what happens during a sexual encounter is determined by what the woman enjoys having done to her, and so she also exerts some control. The man may also be in a position to derive feelings of achievement, or "conquest," from sex, but his approaching it as a performance also stands in the way of his ability to experience sex on an emotional level, as a means of achieving intimacy with another person.

As discussed in chapter 1, their sexual scripts tend to press men and women to achieve sexual arousal mainly through certain channels. By following his sexual script, the man has relatively little opportunity to experience sexual arousal in the same way his partner does (having his body touched in pleasant ways). And because they have few such opportunities, men seldom develop the same sort of sexual awareness of their bodies that women do.

Helping you make a start in the direction of a new sexual awareness is the purpose of the next exercise.

Exercise 2.5: Exploring Yourself
Do this exercise when you will have forty-five minutes to one hour of uninterrupted privacy.

Begin by taking a leisurely shower. Wash yourself, and then just stand beneath the shower for awhile and concentrate on the way your body feels as the water hits it in different places. Move slowly around so that the spray hits various spots on your body: head, face, and neck; shoulders, back, and chest; buttocks, genitals, thighs, legs, and feet. Notice how the stimulation feels in each of these places. Try changing the water temperature a little, and, if you can, adjust the spray so that it is harder or softer. Take your time. When you feel ready to stop, towel off, slowly and not roughly. As you do this, notice how the different parts of your body feel as you run your towel across them.

When you are completely dry, stand in front of a mirror, a full-length one if possible. Spend about fifteen minutes going over your body carefully. Look at yourself from head to toe in the mirror. Try not to skip anything. This may feel uncomfortable but try to stay with it. Look closely at your hair, your face (eyes, nose, cheeks, mouth, chin), your neck, shoulders, and arms. Look at each of your hands (front and back) and at your fingers. Then look at your chest. Watch yourself breathe. Next, look at your stomach, closely, then your thighs, your legs, and your feet. Look at your toes. Now, stand up straight and look at your genitals in the mirror. Look at them, don't look away. See your penis, your pubic hair, and your scrotum. Turn to the side and look at your genitals in profile. Notice the size, shape, color, and texture of things.

Put on your robe now and get into bed. Lie down, but prop your back up with something, perhaps a couple of pillows. Open or remove your robe, and start to look at your body close up for a second time. Look at your arms, hands, chest, and stomach. Look at each one of your fingers and at your wrists. Look down at your legs, feet, and toes. Then look at your genitals. When you are finished looking, slowly begin to explore your body with your hands. Start by using a light touch and soft, stroking movements. Explore your head, face, and neck first, thoroughly, and then your arms, hands, and chest. Take a minute to stroke your stomach lightly and experience how it feels. Then do the same with your thighs (inside and out). Then roll over on your stomach and stroke your buttocks and your back (as much as you can reach). Finish by touching your legs, feet, and toes. Again, take your time. Notice, as you explore yourself, how sensitive your whole body is to touch and how much potential it has for pleasure.

Now touch your genitals. Run your fingers gently through your pubic hair and note its length and texture. Notice also the way that kind of stroking feels. Touch your penis next, noting the texture of its skin and the way it feels when it is stroked. Look at the glans of your penis (pulling back the foreskin if you are not circumsized) and the shaft. Stroke the glans lightly with your finger tips and notice the sensitivity. See if there are places on the glans that are more sensitive than others. Take your penis in your fingers and stroke it gently several times. Notice how good the sensations in your penis can be. If it begins to get erect, watch and feel this happening as you continue stroking yourself lightly. Last of all, explore your scrotum. Note whether its skin at the moment is loose or taut and how it feels when you stroke it lightly. Press lightly, so that you can trace the outlines of your testes inside the scrotum. Then, when you feel ready to stop, lie back, cover yourself if you feel cool, and relax for ten minutes or so. Try to clear your mind of thoughts and concentrate on breathing easily and deeply.

How did you react to this exercise? Were you embarrassed to look at your own body, even though you were completely alone? If so, what sort of attitude toward yourself do you suppose that sort of reaction might reflect? Were you very critical of your body, or did you find parts that you think are attractive and pleasant to look at? Was it more difficult to look at or touch your genitals than other parts of your body?

In order for you to begin really appreciating the erotic potential of your whole body, you should do this exercise more than once, preferably several times. You may need to get past an initial awkward stage, in which you find the exercise embarrassing or silly, before you can begin experiencing your body without such interfering reactions. If you become sexually aroused and want to finish the exercise by masturbating to orgasm, or by inviting your partner to have a sexual encounter, do so. However, make sure that you do the actual exercise alone, and make sure also that you give yourself enough time so that you do not have to rush through it. Your schedule may be busy, but you owe yourself the time. This is important learning you are doing here.

Once you begin to experience the pleasure that your body can give you, you will appreciate more and more your own sexual sensitivities. You really are sensitive; it is simply a matter of discovering the fact. You also have unique sexual preferences—places and ways you like being touched best, which are unique to you. If you want to, you can begin to use your sexual sensitivities and the entire erotic potential of your own body in your sexual encounters by switching roles with your partner and asking her to make love to you. This would involve both of you breaking free of your sexual scripts, which may not be an easy thing to do at first, but you both stand to gain a lot if you take that risk.

SUMMARY

The goal of this chapter is to help you begin the process of liberating yourself from outdated and limiting ideas about your sexuality by exploring your individuality. By focusing attention on factors that relate to your sexual interest and on the erotic potential of your body, you may have been able to discover two things. The first basic idea is that you do have sexual sensitivities. Your sexual interests, for example, are not purely instinct; they are heavily influenced by circumstances. Some of the factors that affect your sexual desire are the physical appearance and character of a particular woman and the nature of your relationship together. If these things are right for you, your sexual desire will be stimulated, and if they are not, your desire will suffer. Similarly, you have a body that is very sexually sensitive; that is, it has a great deal of erotic potential that can be developed, if you are willing to commit the time and effort necessary to doing so.

The second discovery you, hopefully, will have made as a result of the exercises in this chapter is that you are not only sexually sensitive, but you have a set of personal preferences that is unique to you as an individual. Again, it may take time and effort to discover something about these preferences, but they are there. You are not, in short. a carbon copy of every other man.

Discovering that you have sexual sensitivities and are a sexually unique individual has implications for your present sexual relationship and your future sexual fulfillment. Once you have made these discoveries, you have a choice of acting on them or not. Not acting will mean that your relationship will remain at its present level, sexually speaking, for both you and your partner. If you are satisfied but feel that you can get even more from your relationship, or if you are not sexually satisfied at present, by all means experiment with acting on the knowledge you have gained in this chapter.

3 enhancing your sexual relationship

The exercises in chapter 2 were designed to help you begin a process of self-discovery and change. Learning more about yourself, and specifically about your individual sexuality, is one way to begin changing your sex life for the better. In that case, you are essentially working on *yourself*. In this chapter, the exercises will help you to begin working on your *relationship*.

Although it is possible to work alone on changing your sexual relationship, efforts to liberate yourself from restrictive sexual patterns are more likely to succeed if you and your partner (or partners) can work together toward this same end. A shared interest in enhancing the quality of your sexual relationship will have the effect of drawing you closer and will make it easier to get through the initial awkward phase that is so often a part of change. If each person is willing to accept some responsibility for the work that is necessary, your chances of success are more than double what they would be if only one of you was interested in changing things. In addition, each of you must be willing, as individuals, to take risks, to push yourself to try new things, and to stick with things through the rough spots. You ought to think about this before beginning, to decide for yourself if you are interested in changing, and it would be valuable as well if you could share with each other your hopes as well as your apprehensions ahead of time. Take the opportunity to do this now, before reading on; it will be well worth the delay.

The exercises in this chapter focus on three different areas, each of which relates directly to the problem of breaking free of old patterns and building new lovemaking skills. The first area concerns *sexual communication,* learning to let your partner know what pleases you and what doesn't, what you want and what you don't want. The second area concerns how to assess your *sexual repertoire,* the things you include (and don't include) as part of your sexual relationship. You will also be guided in directions that will help you to begin developing new lovemaking patterns. The third area involves giving some thought to the task of establishing a *sexual situation,* an atmosphere that will be conducive to pleasure.

Once again, although these exercises have been designed by a man, for men, your sexual partner may find them equally useful. Especially because of the fact that sexual fulfillment is best accomplished when it is a shared goal, approached as a joint responsibility, it is recommended that your partner at least read through the exercises even if she prefers not to do them herself.

SEXUAL COMMUNICATION

Broadly speaking, there are two kinds of communication you need to make effectively in sexual situations. The first is to communicate what you like and want, and the second is to communicate what you don't like and to let it be known when you don't want something. The first type of communication has to do with sharing *positive* feelings and the second has to do with sharing *negative* feelings. The more you are able to communicate your feelings effectively, both positive and negative, the more likely you are to maximize your personal preferences and minimize sources of discomfort during a sexual encounter. Personal experience as a sex therapist has led to the feeling that improved sexual communication, in and of itself, can lead directly to greater sexual fulfillment for many couples. Communication can be either *verbal* or *nonverbal*. That is, people can communicate positive and negative feelings using *words* or *gestures*. If you would like your partner to touch your body in a certain place and in a specific way, you can either ask her (verbal communication) or show her (nonverbal communication), for instance, by putting her hand where you want it or by showing her by touching yourself first. Similarly, if you don't like to be touched in a particular place or in a certain way, you can either ask your partner to do something else, or you can take her hand away, or show her what you would like better. In this section we will explore both verbal and nonverbal ways of communicating.

In one specific area, you may already be an effective sexual communicator, and that is in communicating to your partner that you would like to have sex with her. Not all men are good at, or feel comfortable with, even this type of sexual communication; but in general men seem to be able to communicate their desire for sexual contact better than they can anything else. This is because, as a man, you have been taught that it is your responsibility to initiate sexual contact. By now you may be so used to this arrangement that you are, or would be, put off by a woman who took direct sexual initiative on her own. Such a situation might seem "unnatural," or you might feel that such a woman was being overly aggressive. What she would actually be doing is simply taking responsibility for initiating what happens between the two of you sexually, but since you are used to having this responsibility yourself, you might feel ill at ease.

Sexual attitudes in our culture are slowly changing; people are beginning to liberate themselves from the need to restrict their lovemaking to the usual sexual scripts. Unfortunately, this change is a slow process, and many men and women still believe that it is strictly a man's place to take the sexual initiative.

Usually, they also believe that the contents of a sexual encounter (who does what to whom) is pretty much the man's responsibility. But when each of two persons shares in the responsibility for what happens between them, he or she is freed from restrictive sexual scripts. When things go well, it is to the credit of the relationship, rather than being one individual's accomplishment. If and when things go poorly, that is a burden to be shared, too, and a problem to be solved together, rather than being simply a reflection of your inadequacy as a man.

A sexual relationship based on shared responsibility requires better communication than one in which only one of the partners has all the responsibility. Aside from being able to communicate their sexual desire, men are no better than women at sexual communication. Believing the myths about male sexuality, and trying their best to follow the sexual script laid out for them, most men never disclose to their partners if they feel unfulfilled in their sexual relationships. Instead, they go elsewhere, or they suffer in silence until they lose interest in sex or develop a sexual dysfunction. Since we are expected to be the active doers in a sexual encounter, it is especially difficult for men to ask to be fondled, touched, or caressed in particular ways. It does not feel "natural" for us to take the passive receiver role and to allow our partners to make love to us. Similarly, the idea of becoming active, of initiating sexual contact or making love to a man, may seem foreign or "unnatural" to many women.

It makes sense that, once you have an awareness of what pleases you sexually, a failure to feel sexually satisfied can be linked to one of three possibilities: you are having sex when you don't really feel like it; you have not communicated your sexual preferences effectively to your partner; or you have communicated effectively, but your wishes have been rejected or ignored. Of these three, the first and second are by far the most common. These problems can be dealt with by improving your ability to communicate. In the first instance, you need to know when you do and do not want sex, and then you need to make your feelings known. In the second instance, you need to communicate your preferences. A technique called *behavioral rehearsal* will be used here. It will help you to overcome your fears about communicating positive and negative feelings in sexual situations, and it will provide you with an opportunity to practice verbal communication.

Exercise 3.1: Fears about Communicating

Sit back and relax for a minute or two. Put the book down, clear your mind of distractions, and concentrate on taking deep breaths. When you feel ready, read the following scenes and try to imagine them happening to you.

SCENE 1
You are in a nice restaurant. You have just finished having dinner with a woman whom you find very sexually appealing. She looks at you and smiles, and then says, "Would you like to come back to my place for awhile?" Reaching out, she gently touches your hand and says, "You really turn me on."

SCENE 2
You are in bed making love, and after kissing and caressing your lover for awhile, you lay back, look at her, and say, "I'd really like it if you made love to me."

SCENE 3
You are lying back in bed, and your partner is making love to you. When she does something that feels good, you groan, sigh, or say how good it feels. You ask her to caress your arms and hands. At one point, she presses down on your arm more firmly than you would like. You take her hand in yours and stroke yourself gently with it for a moment until she gets the message.

Do the above scenes seem "real" or "unreal" to you? Do they describe something you do often? Do you think you might feel a little up-tight in one or another of these situations?

Scene 1 illustrates a woman taking responsibility for initiating sexual contact. This is not the typical pattern taught to us in our culture, and many men would feel tense or put off to some extent in this situation. In Scene 2, you imagine yourself asking to be made love to, which means taking a passive receiver role during a lovemaking session. Scene 3 illustrates fairly clear sexual communication on your part during a sexual encounter, while you are in the passive receiver role. This, too, is not typical. Most men seldom leave the active doer role, and even when they do, they do not generally do much talking or asking for things. Since these scenes are unusual, any or all of them may seem "unnatural" to you. Of course, nature has nothing to do with it; our usual patterns of lovemaking are just habits that become so strong, they eventually *seem* natural.

You may agree that it would be nice to be able to share responsibility, for you as a man to be able to take the passive receiver role at times, and to be able to communicate openly during a sexual encounter. If so, you have made an important decision, and these things may now be goals for you. As you no doubt know, however, setting a goal is not the same thing as reaching it. If you are not used to doing the sorts of things described in the three scenes, it is very likely that you will feel tense or nervous if and when you first try them out. This tension may have been evident already in your reactions to imagining the scenes. For instance, as you read them, you may have felt your stomach tighten up just a little or your face become flushed. A response of tension in such situations is often linked to two fears. The first is a fear of rejection. If you have never before asked to be made love to, talked out loud while making love, or told a lover that something she is doing makes you uncomfortable, one reason may be that you would expect a negative reaction if you did.

A second fear often linked to a tension response is that you will not be able to do it right if you try something new, for instance, ask to be made love to. This is a fear of awkwardness, which is also linked to the traditional male sexual scripts and myths about male sexuality. Since men feel they ought to be experts when it comes to sex, the idea of being awkward ("like a beginner") is embarrassing. In our culture it has (at least in the past) been acceptable for a woman to say that she is not very sexually experienced, but chances are that a man would be embarrassed to admit such a thing. This need to be, or at least to seem to be, a sexual expert is a trap for men. It is probably the main reason why any twenty-one-year-old virgin man would be terribly embarrassed to admit that he has not yet had sexual intercourse, and it is also the reason why you would be afraid to try out something new during a sexual encounter. It is, even more generally, the reason why most men are so sensitive to criticism, direct or implied, about their sexual skills. They believe that they should know what turns a woman on and be able to do it. It never occurs to them that what turns one woman on might not work with another, and that they, therefore, need to learn something about each lover they have. Instead, they believe that all women like the same sorts of things, just as women believe that all men like the same sorts of things. Men don't think of women as having individual sexualities any more than they think of themselves that way, or any more than women think of men that way.

Most men have not had ten, twenty, or thirty lovers, and most men have not tried everything under the sun in the way of sexual activities. Neither are men able to read a woman's mind and know what she likes without receiving some sort of message. Yet many men act as if they should be able to do these things.

Despite the fact that we live in an age of so-called sexual freedom or openness, the pressures on men to be sexual experts seem to be getting greater, not less, forcing men to be less open about themselves sexually. This pressure is reflected, for example, in men's magazines, where, if you believe the letters and columns, the world is overflowing with Casanovas. Hard-core pornography is even worse. These magazines and films encourage ridiculously unrealistic expectations for men and women alike. In these fairy tales, men are depicted as sexual machines who are such expert lovers that women are beating down the doors to get at them. They can turn on and satisfy any woman, anytime, anyplace; and their sexual performance is always the same—perfect. The only potentially positive aspect of these fantasies seems to be that in them the man does sometimes take the passive receiver role, and women are viewed as having independent sex drives. This seems also to be the basis of their appeal. More often than not, however, there is little in the way of sexual communication depicted in pornographic sex, and this is most unfortunate, for we are expected to believe in men and women who are sexually identical, having the same likes and few, if any, dislikes.

Pornography is not reality, but men frequently act as if it were. They do so by striving to be like the males in the magazines and movies. In doing so, men set themselves up to feel like failures when they cannot meet these unrealistic expectations. One man, for instance, was astounded to see that the man in one film I showed him did not have an erection, despite the fact that he was making love to an attractive woman, who, at one point, stimulated his genitals with her mouth and tongue. He really believed that there was something wrong with this man, when, in fact, it was obvious that the man in the film was tense, probably because of the filming situation. In this particular instance, the viewer's reactions illustrate the destructiveness of myths about male sexuality: expecting yourself to perform like a sexual machine is self-defeating.

Men close themselves off to new possibilities for pleasure when they are afraid to seem like beginners, when, in fact, they are beginners. Because they think they ought to know, instinctively, what pleases a woman, they hesitate to ask what pleases her. Because they are not sure if some new position might be comfortable or uncomfortable, they don't suggest trying it, and so on.

Experience as a sex therapist has convinced me that shared responsibility and open communication lead to better, more fulfilling sex for both partners. More than that, these things generally tend to affect the quality of a relationship in a positive way, making it more meaningful and intimate. To work toward such goals, you will need to confront your anxiety about changing. This means, first of all, accepting the fact that you are likely to be nervous trying something new. You will never know for sure, until you've tried it, just how your partner will react to something or whether you will like it yourself. In lovemaking as in anything else, skill comes only with practice, patience, and persistence. Expecting yourself to do anything perfectly the first time is a losing proposition. There is no exercise that will truly substitute for actual experience in real situations. The best that exercises can do is to offer you a way of breaking the ice. Following through with these exercises, as they are written, may help reduce both your anxiety and awkwardness when the time does come to experiment with changes in a real relationship, but they are not likely to eliminate the awkward phase.

Exercise 3.2: Learning to Communicate

Sit back and relax for a minute. Put the book down, clear your mind, and take some easy, deep breaths. When you feel ready, go on.

In each of the following scenes, you will be asked to experiment with saying some things to an imaginary woman. This technique is called behavioral rehearsal. The notion behind it is that if you practice saying things to an imaginary woman, it might be a little easier, and less awkward, to do so later on with a real woman. The technique works, and it works best if you practice your lines *out loud*. Therefore, it is best if you do this exercise in a private place where you can talk out loud without feeling embarrassed.

SCENE 1

Imagine that you are in a restaurant with a woman you like very much. It is your first date together. Take a minute or two to create this scene in your mind's eye. Give the woman a face, a voice, a body, clothes, and even a name. Picture the restaurant, your own table, the people around you. In short, make your imaginary woman, and the situation, seem as real as you possibly can. Now, try saying the following lines, out loud, *to this imaginary woman: "I find you very attractive. I enjoy being with you."*

Say the lines again, out loud. Imagine the woman in front of you, yourself looking at her, as you say them.

Try the lines again, but this time change the words slightly while getting the same message across.

How did that feel? Were you tense? Don't be too concerned if it seemed odd to be talking to an imaginary woman. Keep in mind the fact that behavioral rehearsal works if you follow through with it. If you were tense while saying the lines the third time, repeat them out loud as many times as necessary until you are able to do it without getting particularly up-tight. Be sure to try imagining that this is a real woman you are saying these things to. When you feel fairly comfortable saying the lines in Scene 1, go on to Scene 2.

SCENE 2

Imagine that you are in your apartment with the same woman you made up in Scene 1. You embrace and kiss, and then you let her go and move back a little. She looks at you curiously. A moment passes, and then she asks you if you are feeling okay. Say to her, out loud: *"I feel fine. But you look as if you don't."*

Imagine that your date frowns a little. Imagine yourself looking at her, and say, out loud: *"Were you expecting me to make some sort of a sexual move just then?"*

Your date smiles, nods, and says that she was sort of hoping that you would make a sexual advance. Say to her, out loud: *"I am very attracted to you, but to be honest I just don't feel ready for a sexual relationship with you yet. I'd really like to see you again and get to know you better. I hope you can understand that."*

Again, make sure that as you go through Scene 2 you picture yourself with a real woman and that you say each of your lines out loud. Go through the whole scene a second time, changing the words to suit yourself while getting the same message across. If you find yourself feeling very tense doing it, repeat the scene a third time.

What sort of reaction would you expect to get from the woman in Scene 2? What would be your worst fear about the way she might react if you said these things? Would she laugh at you? Think you weren't normal? What would be your response to that? Would you feel ashamed? How would you like a woman to react if you said these sorts of things to her?

Chances are if you expected a bad reaction to Scene 2, and if you think that kind of reaction would make you feel bad, you will be nervous about it until you have an opportunity to try this sort of thing in a real-life situation. Most likely you will discover that if a woman likes you and wants to have a relationship with you, she will be able to accept this sort of limit-setting on your part. In fact, you may be surprised to discover that some women will be relieved that you don't expect them to go to bed with you on your first date. There is no guarantee that you won't encounter a woman who does react negatively when you tell her that you like her, but don't want to go to bed with her on your first or second date, especially if she does want to. However, if you don't want to go to bed quickly, you are most likely interested in having a relationship, not recreational sex (see chapter 2), whereas a woman who would reject your limit-setting is probably less interested in having a relationship with you.

When you feel reasonably comfortable doing the Scene 2 exercises, proceed to Scene 3.

SCENE 3

Imagine that you are in bed with your imaginary lover and that you are making love to her. Imagine that, initially you are in the active doer role and that she is in the passive receiver role. Picture yourself touching her body, making love to her. Say to her, out loud *and* softly: *"Does that feel good?"*

Repeat the line again, out loud and softly.

Now, with the same scene in mind, say to your lover, out loud and gently: "I'd really like it if you would tell me what feels good when I'm touching you."

Say the line again, changing the words slightly if you like.

Imagine again this same lovemaking scene. Say to your lover: "I'd like to think that you'd tell me if there was anything I'm doing that you don't really like. I want to please you."

Repeat the line, and then repeat the entire exercise once more before moving on.

After pleasing your partner in an active way for a while, imagine that you kiss her and say, out loud: *"I'd like it if you would touch me for a while."*

Repeat this last line, out loud and gently, several times. You can change the words to suit yourself, but get the same message across. You want to be able to say the words—that is, make the request to be made love to—without a lot of nervous tension. Once you are able to do this, pay attention to your voice. You want to be gentle, yet you want to get your message across. When you feel you can do this fairly well, move on to the next paragraph.

Imagine yourself lying back while your partner caresses you. Imagine that she touches you somewhere in a way that you find very pleasant. Say to her, out loud: *"That feels good."*

Practice this simple statement, and others like it, several times, until you feel you are able to communicate pleasure fairly easily, without a lot of nervousness. Then move on.

Imagine that you are being made love to and are enjoying it, but that you would also like some particular kind of stimulation that your partner hasn't given you yet. Say to her, out loud: *"That feels good. I'd like it if you would (whatever it is you might like), if you'd like to."*

Repeat these lines, changing the words a little if you like, several times. Practice being able to make a sexual request without feeling up-tight about it. Then pay some attention to your voice. Do you sound angry, critical? If you do, your attitude might put off your lover. Remember, you can't expect her to know all your preferences without being told. It is always nice to be appreciated, and telling her what feels good can make it easier for your partner to accept a request without feeling criticized. Finally, keep in mind the possibility that she might turn down your request. That would not mean that you were wrong to ask, or that your own preferences are bad in any way. When you feel ready, move on to the next paragraph.

> *Imagine that your lover asks you to do something to her that you don't particularly enjoy doing. Say to her,* out loud: *"I'm sorry, but I really don't want to do that. Is there something else I can do for you instead?"*

Be sure to say your lines out loud. Repeat them until you can do so without feeling embarrassed or guilty about saying no. Then pay attention to the way in which you are saying no. Do you sound scolding, disapproving? Remember that people are as different in their sexual tastes as they are in their preferences about anything else. You have the right to decline to do things that are not to your own tastes, but you ought not to assume that someone else's preferences are bad just because they are different from yours. Turning down a sexual request can be a difficult thing for a man to do. You would be wise, therefore, to practice this particular part of the exercise several times, using different variations to get the same message across. Then move on.

> *Imagine that your partner is stimulating you in a way that she seems to like, but that you don't. Say to her,* out loud: *"I am not sure I like that as much as you do. I think I'd like it better if you (whatever would please you better) instead."*

Repeat these lines, out loud, several times. Aim first at being able to say them without feeling tense. Second, pay some attention to how your voice sounds. Once again, work at getting your message across without being unduly rough about it. After all, you really have to be firm only if you have already communicated the same message clearly several times, and you are still ignored. Remember that you cannot expect your lover to know what you are feeling by reading your mind, and that sometimes people do forget things.

In sexual situations clear, but gentle and caring, communication seems to work best. People are especially sensitive in such situations, and you want to be sure to treat your lover the way you would like her to treat you. However, personal sensitivity is no reason to avoid communicating. Even though it may be difficult at first, work on it; you stand to gain a great deal.

It might be a good idea for you to repeat all of Exercise 3.2 at least twice, perhaps several times, if you feel especially uptight about sexual communication. Each time, try your best to imagine the scenes clearly, making them as real as possible in your own mind, and remember to say your lines out loud. Doing this should make it easier for you to begin communicating in real sexual situations. However, remember that there is no real substitute for actual experience. Even if you are able to do the above behavioral rehearsals well, expect yourself to make a mistake or two or at least to be a bit awkward in a real situation, the first few times you try to communicate verbally. Be a little tolerant with yourself. Most of all, think about your sexual self-image as a man. Do you expect yourself to be a sexual expert, who can do things flawlessly the first time around, or can you think of yourself as a human being, who is not perfect and can only learn from experience?

Nonverbal Communication

So far in this section we have worked mainly on overcoming fears of communication and on developing skills in *verbal* communication. But words are only one way of getting a message across to another person. A second way, as mentioned earlier, is through nonverbal communication, which includes, among other things, showing someone what you want or don't want.

When you learn to communicate your sexual preferences by showing someone rather than telling them, you are learning to *model* your preferences. Modeling is an especially effective way of learning; under certain circumstances it is more effective than words. Particularly in the case of learning a skill, be it lovemaking or building a cabinet, having someone show you what to do rather than just telling you speeds the learning process considerably. Modeling is, in a sense, a more direct way of learning. Improving your ability to communicate nonverbally can be a great asset to your sexual relationship. For two people, learning to give one another pleasure is a skill that does not come naturally but needs to be developed over time.

Communicating sexual preferences nonverbally can be effectively accomplished by showing your partner how to pleasure you, and by her doing likewise. The following guidelines can be helpful in getting you started on communicating nonverbally.

- You can ask your partner to take your hand in hers and stroke herself with it in a way that she finds pleasing. In that way you can learn directly what kind of touch she prefers and where she likes to be touched best.
- You can put your hand over your partners while she touches herself in a way that she likes.
- You can ask your partner to stimulate herself while you watch the way she does it.
- You can have your partner put her hand over yours while you stimulate yourself in a way that pleases you.
- You can put your hand over your partners while she stimulates you, and you can guide her in terms of where and how to touch you.
- You can stimulate yourself while your partner watches the way you do it.

In reading the above list, you may be able to see how important it is for you to develop an awareness of your own body. By learning more about your body, about what pleases you, you will be in a better position to communicate your desires to your partner. If you have not as yet done it, Exercise 2.5 (Exploring Yourself) in chapter 2 will be useful.

Although the above guidelines give some hints about how to begin communicating nonverbally, you must expect it to take some time for you to develop effective nonverbal communication skills in your relationship. Much of your learning will involve trial and error. The most difficult phase will occur when you first begin to experiment. If both you and your partner are motivated to improve your sexual communication, this initial awkward stage will be shorter than if only one of you is trying. Don't expect yourselves to do it right immediately. You may feel uncomfortable the first few times, as you do whenever you try something new.

If you tend to be sexually inhibited, as many people are, you may find nonverbal communication embarrassing at first. Again, getting started will be the most difficult part. After a while, your embarrassment should subside, allowing your comfort and sexual pleasure to increase. It helps, too, if you can share your awkwardness or embarrassment with your partner, and she with you. Being able to encourage one another and give each other sympathy and support can go a long way toward getting through difficulties. Finally, learning to laugh together when you feel awkward or embarrassed will be extremely helpful when you are in the midst of learning your new lovemaking skills.

EXPANDING SEXUAL REPERTOIRES

Your sexual repertoire refers to the number and variety of different sexual activities that are part of your sexual relationship. A couple could be said to have a *narrow* sexual repertoire if in their sexual relationship they typically engage in only a few different activities. This would contrast with a *broad* sexual repertoire, characterized by a couple who typically engage in many different activities during their sexual encounters. Finally, a couple can have either a *balanced* or an *unbalanced* sexual repertoire, depending on how much each partner gets and gives in the sexual relationship. If each partner seems to get about as much as he or she gives, then the sexual relationship could be said to be balanced; otherwise, it is unbalanced to a greater or lesser extent.

Couples can benefit from working toward making their sexual repertoire both broad and balanced. That is not to say that each and every sexual encounter should be this way. Sometimes a sexual encounter can be limited to just a few activities, and it can still be extremely satisfying to both partners. And there certainly can be times when one partner only gives and the other only gets, which can also be extremely satisfying. However if, over the long run, a sexual relationship is narrow and/or unbalanced, chances are high that one or both partners will eventually feel sexually unfulfilled.

The purpose of this section is, first, to help you assess your sexual repertoire, to determine whether it is broad or narrow, balanced or unbalanced. The second purpose is to provide you with directions to pursue in order to broaden and/or balance your sexual repertoire.

Exercise 3.3: Your Sexual Repertoire

For this exercise, you will need about an hour, plus two pencils or pens in different colors. The instructions assume that you will be using blue and red although, of course, you may substitute others. You will also need the Sexual Activity Checklist and the Sexual Activity Coding Sheet, on the following pages. The exercise is to be done in two parts.

PART 1

Go through the Sexual Activity Checklist slowly and carefully. Note that each activity listed has a number and that these numbers appear on the Sexual Activity Coding Sheet as well. There are a total of 33 specific sexual activities, plus several blank spaces you can use to add any additional activities. For each activity listed, indicate a pleasure *rating on the Sexual Activity Coding Sheet. (Do this in red.) The pleasure rating should reflect how much you enjoy a particular activity (or, if you've never tried it, how much you think you might enjoy it). Use the system below to assign a pleasure rating to each activity on the checklist.*

Pleasure Rating	Meaning
1	Extremely unpleasurable for you
2	Moderately unpleasurable for you
3	Mildly unpleasurable for you
4	Mildly pleasurable for you
5	Moderately pleasurable for you
6	Extremely pleasurable for you

When assigning pleasure ratings, make sure that the rating is for the right activity number. Complete all pleasure ratings before going on to Part 2.

SEXUAL ACTIVITY CHECKLIST

Activity	Description of Sexual Activity
1	Seeing your partner naked
2	Being seen naked by your partner
3	Holding your partner in your arms
4	Being held in your partner's arms
5	Kissing each other on the lips
6	Stroking or caressing your partner's body through her clothing
7	Your partner caressing your body through your clothes
8	Kissing your partner using your tongue
9	Your partner kissing you using her tongue
10	Stroking or caressing your partner's naked body all over
11	Your partner caressing your naked body all over

Activity (cont.)	Description of Sexual Activity (cont.)
12	Caressing your partner's naked body all over using your mouth, lips, and tongue
13	Your partner caressing your naked body all over using her mouth, lips, and tongue
14	Kissing or sucking your partner's breasts
15	Your partner kissing or sucking your breasts
16	Caressing or stroking your partner's genitals with your hands
17	Your partner caressing your genitals with her hands
18	Caressing your partner's genitals with your mouth, lips, and tongue
19	Your partner caressing your genitals with her mouth, lips, and tongue
20	Stroking your partner's genitals with your hands until she reaches orgasm (climax)
21	Your partner caressing your genitals with her hands until you reach orgasm (climax)
22	Caressing your partner's genitals using your mouth until she reaches orgasm
23	Your partner caressing your genitals using her mouth until you reach orgasm
24	Stimulating your partner's body with a vibrator
25	Your partner stimulating your body with a vibrator
26	Stimulating your partner's genitals with a vibrator until she reaches orgasm
27	Your partner stimulating your genitals with a vibrator until you reach orgasm
28	Having intercourse with you on top and your partner under you
29	Having intercourse with your partner on top
30	Having intercourse with you and your partner lying side to side and face to face
31	Having intercourse from the rear (with your partner lying on her stomach or on all fours)
32	Having intercourse from the rear while lying side to side
33	Having intercourse with both of you in a sitting position
34	_____
35	_____

SEXUAL ACTIVITY CODING SHEET

Each activity is identified by number on the Sexual Activity Checklist. Go through the Checklist and assign each activity a pleasure rating (using blue). Then go through the Checklist a second time and assign each activity a frequency rating (using red).

Activity

	1	2	3	4	5	6	7	8	9	10	11	12	13	14	15	16	17	18	19	20	21	22	23	24	25	26	27	28	29	30	31	32	33	34	35
	1	1	1	1	1	1	1	1	1	1	1	1	1	1	1	1	1	1	1	1	1	1	1	1	1	1	1	1	1	1	1	1	1	1	1
	2	2	2	2	2	2	2	2	2	2	2	2	2	2	2	2	2	2	2	2	2	2	2	2	2	2	2	2	2	2	2	2	2	2	2
	3	3	3	3	3	3	3	3	3	3	3	3	3	3	3	3	3	3	3	3	3	3	3	3	3	3	3	3	3	3	3	3	3	3	3
	4	4	4	4	4	4	4	4	4	4	4	4	4	4	4	4	4	4	4	4	4	4	4	4	4	4	4	4	4	4	4	4	4	4	4
	5	5	5	5	5	5	5	5	5	5	5	5	5	5	5	5	5	5	5	5	5	5	5	5	5	5	5	5	5	5	5	5	5	5	5
	6	6	6	6	6	6	6	6	6	6	6	6	6	6	6	6	6	6	6	6	6	6	6	6	6	6	6	6	6	6	6	6	6	6	6

Pleasure/Frequency Rating

PART 2

Go through the Sexual Activity Checklist a second time, this time giving each activity a frequency rating. *(Do this in blue.) Put the frequency ratings on the Coding Sheet, making sure that you are rating the correct activity each time by checking its number. The frequency rating is a measure of how often each activity usually occurs when you have a sexual encounter. Imagine the last several times you have had an encounter, and then indicate how often, on the average, each activity was a part of those encounters. Use the system below to assign these ratings.*

Frequency Rating	Meaning
1	Never or almost never happens during your sexual encounters
2	Very seldom happens (about once in every ten encounters)
3	Sometimes happens (two or three times in ten encounters)
4	Often happens (four to six times in ten encounters)
5	Very often happens (six to nine times in ten encounters)
6	Always or almost always happens during your sexual encounters

Now that you have gone through the Sexual Activity Checklist twice, giving each activity listed a pleasure rating and then a frequency rating, take some time to study the results on your Coding Sheet. Take note first of those sexual activities you say turn you on most (those that have pleasure ratings of 5 and 6). Note what they are and whether they are mostly things you like to have done to you, mostly things you enjoy doing to your partner, or whether your preferences include activities of both types.

If you mainly enjoy things that are done to you, you may discover that your partner does not feel that she is getting as much as she is giving in your sexual encounters, which in turn will affect how sexually fulfilling your relationship is for her. Some men have a sort of negative reaction to women's bodies. They may, for instance, not like to touch or look at a woman's genitals. This tendency will usually be reflected in many low pleasure ratings among activities 1, 3, 5, 8, 10, 12, 14, 16, 18, 20, 22, 24, and 26. This sort of fear of women is not uncommon, but, if you have it, it is one you might seriously consider trying to overcome. (Chapter 8 deals with this issue.)

Look through your Coding Sheet again. This time check out those activities that are usually a part of your sexual encounters (those with frequency ratings of 4, 5, and 6). Are there many of them or just a few? Often people report an increased sense of sexual fulfillment when they work toward expanding their sexual repertoire, that is, broadening it. You can identify some likely target for such experimenting by searching through your Coding Sheet for places where your pleasure rating and frequency rating for a particular activity are far apart. Normally, you would expect that if a person did not enjoy a sexual activity, he or she would not do it very often. Consequently, the more you enjoy an activity, the more often you would expect it to occur. Ideally, then, your pleasure ratings and frequency ratings should be fairly close. Look for places where your pleasure rating is high (5 or 6), but the frequency rating is low (1, 2, or 3). These are sexual activities you say you enjoy, or think you would enjoy, but which do not happen very often. These are the activities you should begin to experiment with in order to expand your sexual repertoire and increase your sense of sexual fulfillment.

Looking through your Coding Sheet a third time will give you some idea as to how balanced your repertoire is, how much psychic stimulation versus direct stimulation (as discussed in chapter 1) you typically get during your sexual encounters. Recall that both of these types of stimulation contribute to your sexual arousal. Check your frequency ratings for sexual activities 4, 7, 9, 11, 13, 15, 17, 19, 21, 23, 25, and 27. Are these sorts of activities that would give you direct stimulation often or seldom a part of your sexual encounter? Add up the frequency ratings for this set of activities and write down the total.

Look now at the frequency ratings you gave to sexual activities 3, 6, 8, 10, 12, 14, 16, 18, 20, 22, 24, and 26. These activities all involve things that you do to your partner, providing her with direct stimulation. At the same time, your experience of her reaction to these activities—the way she looks, the way she moves, the sounds she makes, and so on—provide you with psychic stimulation. Add up your frequency ratings for this set of activities and write down the total. Compare this number to the total involving direct stimulation of you by your partner. If these two numbers are almost equal, that means that giving and getting are present in about equal parts during your sexual encounters. In short, your sexual repertoire is balanced. Your own sexual arousal, and that of your partner in this case, comes from direct and psychic stimulation in about equal proportions.

If one of these numbers is much higher than the other, you are getting one form of stimulation (psychic or direct) more than the other and so is your partner. If you were to work on increasing the frequency of those activities that contribute to the lower number, you would be developing an additional source of sexual arousal for yourself and your partner. Usually the psychic stimulation figure is higher than the direct stimulation figure for men; the opposite is usually the case for women. If this describes your relationship, you might want to work toward changing this arrangement so that you get more direct stimulation and your partner more psychic stimulation. Exercises 3.1 and 3.2 in this chapter should help you build skills that will enable you to get started in this direction.

The last thing to look for in your Coding Sheet are places where your pleasure rating is low, but the frequency rating is high. These are activities you say you don't enjoy, but which you engage in anyway. Persisting in such a pattern is self-defeating. It will almost invariably lead to feelings of resentment, disgust, or anger, and eventually to a strong dislike of sex. If these activities tend to be ones associated with a fear of women, as described earlier, you will do well to work on that problem.

Remember that the purpose of this section is not to encourage you, or your partner, to become a sexual acrobat. It is based, rather, on the simple notion that there is something to be gained from broadening and balancing sexual repertoires. This is not the same thing as saying that you must be willing to try anything in order to be sexually fulfilled. There is nothing wrong with experimenting—with trying out something new just to see how it feels. By the same token, there is nothing wrong with saying that you don't like something and would just as soon not include it as part of your sexual repertoire.

You and your partner should approach the issue of changing your sexual repertoire as a goal you can pursue in a relaxed manner, not as a demand that you must meet. Give yourselves time to change, trying out perhaps one new thing at a time, just to see if you like it. Use your sexual communication skills to help you. Also, you will be more likely to succeed if you both feel that you each stand to gain something from changing (which is usually the case), and if you both feel some responsibility for this. Probably the worst thing either of you can do is to take all the responsibility for change on your shoulders, or to chastise yourself or the other person for what you have not done in the past.

THE SEXUAL SITUATION

Now it is time to give some thought to the kinds of physical situations you find most conducive to your own sexual enjoyment. This, like all the other things you have been asked to work on, boils down to a matter of personal taste. According to sexual myths, men are not supposed to be very fussy about the setting in which sexual encounters take place; a park bench or telephone booth is as good as a king-size bed in a Riviera resort.

The situation is, therefore, a factor that men (and women) frequently ignore, but it can influence the quality of a sexual encounter a great deal. The sexual script we learn as adolescents is not very detailed in this regard. We learn only that sex should take place in a private, dimly lit place. This probably reflects the attitude our culture has taken toward sex—it is something to be done in secret.

In reality, men do have individual preferences concerning the sexual situation, and the physical setting in which a sexual encounter takes place does influence both their level of sexual arousal and their sexual satisfaction. When the situation pleases them, men will feel more sexually fulfilled by an encounter than they will if the situation is wrong. In fact, if the situation is wrong enough, they may not be able to experience sexual arousal at all.

Some men feel that they get most sexually aroused and enjoy sex the most in the morning when they are rested and the cares of the previous day are behind them; others don't feel turned on at all in the morning, but prefer sex late at night. Some men like sex best in a secluded place, but in the open air; others prefer a bedroom and a locked door. Some men like lots of light; others enjoy darkness. Some like music, incense, special clothing, and mirrors; others don't and so on, and so on. There is no accounting for what is responsible for these differences in personal tastes, and it doesn't really matter. What is important is that you appreciate the fact that circumstances matter, and that you become aware of your own situational preferences so that you can begin to work toward meeting them more fully.

Exercise 3.4: Your Preferred Sexual Situation

Once more, give yourself the time necessary to do this exercise properly. A frequent response men have to my questions is that they haven't spent much time thinking about the sorts of things I ask them. This may be true for you and you might find it difficult at first to come up with answers. Be patient; stick with it. If you do find it frustrating, put the exercise aside for a day or two while you mull it over, and then come back to it.

Go through the following Sexual Situation Chart slowly and carefully. For each area listed, write a description of your personal preferences, specifically your first and second preferences. "Preferences" means a description of what conditions you like, or think you would like, best and second best. They are conditions that you think facilitate or help your sexual arousal and contribute to your sexual enjoyment. For example, under Timing, a man's first preference for sex might be in the morning and a second preference for sex in the early evening. That means that he thinks sex is generally most enjoyable when it happens in the morning and second most when it occurs early in the evening.

SEXUAL SITUATION CHART

For each area, list your first and second preferences. Then assign an importance rating.

Area	First Preference	Second Preference	Importance
Timing: At what time(s) of the day do you prefer to have sex?			1 2
Location: Where do you prefer to have sex?			1 2
Lighting: What kind of lighting do you prefer?			1 2
Decor: What are your preferences for the way the location should look?			1 2
Surface: What kind of surface (bed, rug) do you prefer?			1 2
Clothing: What kind of			

Area	First Preference	Second Preference	Importance
clothing do *you* like to wear?			1 2
Clothing: What kind of clothing do you like your *partner* to wear?			1 2
Other: Music, smell, etc. (Specify _____ _____)			1 2

Next to the preferences you write for each area, assign an importance rating *to that area and to those preferences as a whole. The importance rating is a measure of just how important your preferences in a particular area seem to be for you. Use the following system to assign ratings.*

Importance Rating *Meaning*

1 *Critical.* If one of your two preferences in this area is not met, you will not enjoy a sexual encounter.

2 *Important But Not Critical.* If one of your preferences in this area is not met, you could enjoy a sexual encounter, but only if your preferences in some other area are met.

For example, a man might write under Lighting that he prefers to have sex either in the dark (first preference) or in very dim light (second preference). If he feels that lighting and these particular preferences are so important that he cannot enjoy a sexual encounter under other circumstances (say, in bright sunlight), he would assign Lighting an importance rating of 1. If he felt that his preference in this area was important, but that if the situation was right in other ways he could still enjoy it even if the lighting was wrong, he would assign Lighting an importance rating of 2.

After you have completed your Sexual Situation Chart, note the number of times, if any, that you have circled 1 in the importance rating column. A rating of 1 means that you have a "critical" condition, a personal preference that just has to be met if you are to enjoy a sexual encounter. Depending on how easy or difficult this preference is to meet, you may or may not be limited by it. Feeling that you can enjoy sex only with the lights off won't be much of a problem so long as your preference is okay with your partner. Changing critical conditions, and becoming more flexible, can be approached in the same way as discussed earlier. The technique to use, if you want to change, is to try focusing on those aspects of the situation that do meet your preferences, while ignoring things that bother you.

Another possible solution is to focus on sources of sexual arousal other than your immediate environment, for example, direct stimulation of your body by your partner, your partner's responses, a sexual fantasy, and so on, and to ignore the physical circumstances entirely. Although it may take some time to learn to do this, this solution appears to work for some people. However, the best solution is to try changing the situation to meet your preferences as much as possible. There are many times when it is simply not possible to ignore something about the situation that bothers you, and in which trying to do so seems self-defeating. If privacy is important and, for example, you are afraid of being walked in on by a child, it would be better to satisfy your need rather than ignore your concern. Putting a lock on the bedroom door is a simple and effective solution to this particular concern. If you are worried about waking the children with your lovemaking, it would be better to make love somewhere in the house where they are *not* likely to hear you than to inhibit yourself or keep worrying. If you would really like to have some light on during sex, try to do something about it.

Some men circle no 1's when going through the chart. They report that they can enjoy a sexual encounter so long as at least some of their situational preferences are met. A sexual encounter that meets many of their situational preferences is definitely more enjoyable than one that does not. In other words, just because a preference isn't critical doesn't mean it isn't important. If none of your situational preferences are met by the circumstances under which a sexual encounter takes place, that fact is likely to detract from your enjoyment. One possible solution then is to turn your attention to some other source of arousal and keep it there. This may work if you can do it, but it seems, again, a much better choice to work toward having sex in situations that better suit your tastes.

SUMMARY

The discussion and exercises in chapter 3 are a logical follow-up to those in chapter 2. Their intent is to enable you to build on your knowledge of your own sexual preferences. Once you have increased your self-awareness, the next step is to bring it to bear on the issue of enhancing your sexual relationship. Learning to communicate effectively, reevaluating your sexual repertoire, and giving some thought to the sexual situation are three ways to approach this. More fulfilling relationships, based on shared responsibility, require better communication skills. This communication, in turn, plus your knowledge of what you really want, can be a help in broadening and balancing your sexual repertoire.

Finally, as you come to appreciate your sexual sensitivities, the idea that the circumstances under which sex takes place are important may make more sense to you. Working thoughtfully and selectively, without undue pressure, toward making changes in each of these areas can appreciably improve the quality of your sexual relationship. This will no doubt not happen overnight and you will need to work together, hopefully at a relaxed, playful pace, to realize your goal of sexual fulfillment. You owe it to yourself to pursue this goal, but you also owe it to yourself to be patient and to focus on what is good, at least as much as you do on what is missing.

> *Love*
>
> *To make,*
> *As in a factory,*
> *Cast in precision determination*
> *For profit and caducity?*
>
> *To make*
> *As in over,*
> *That is to fashion the other*
> *Into your own secret image?*
>
> *Or as in do,*
> *To settle for,*
> *Which is always less?*
> *Or as in believe?*
>
> *Perhaps*
> *Not made at all,*
> *But crafted by eccentric motions*
> *And swept by knobbed and muddy hands.*
> ARTHUR DOBRIN

4 developing your sexuality further

Discovering more about your sexuality (chapter 2) and starting to work together with your partner to enhance your sexual relationship (chapter 3) form the foundation of changes that lead to sexual fulfillment. If you have seriously directed yourself toward working on these earlier exercises, especially those in chapter 3, you will have started this process of change. As we have stressed, change is a *process,* not a sudden, all-or-nothing sort of thing. It takes time and persistence, as well as a good measure of patience, to realize the goals you and your partner may have for yourselves and your relationship. You should be thinking in terms of months, not days or weeks, in order to reach these goals.

In this chapter we turn to the issue of developing your sexuality in yet other directions. It is doubtful that any one book could cover all of the ways in which it is possible to explore and develop our sexuality, and for this reason you should spend some time, now and then, browsing through bookstores for volumes that cover areas not included here. In other words, develop an interest in this subject and give yourself permission to pursue it, whether that be through reading, attending lectures or workshops, or taking courses, for example, in sexuality or massage. We live in a time when it is possible (if you want to and if you push yourself a little) to break through the old taboos about sexuality and to explore its possibilities. Several of the topics in this chapter are important areas for beginners to start exploring and developing in order to experience a greater sense of sexual fulfillment.

LETTING YOURSELF BE SEXUAL

We live in a culture in which the expression of sexuality has always been subject to severe constraints. Part of these constraints consist of standards and regulations of behavior: with whom we may have sexual contact and where and when a sexual encounter may properly take place. In addition, in the course of growing up we all develop certain general attitudes toward sex. Although we actually do learn these attitudes, no one has to talk to us directly in order for us to pick them up. We learn them by looking and listening. We notice not only what we see and hear, but also what we don't see and don't hear. Most of all, we watch our parents or other authority figures, and what we see going on between them is taken, for better or worse, as a model for our own adulthood.

It would be rare for a young child in our culture to be aware that his or her parents have a sexual relationship, much less to know the specifics of what they do together or when they make love. Children may (in fact, usually do) have their suspicions, but little or nothing is openly acknowledged. Frequently, sex is not an acceptable topic of conversation within the family and some children never have an opportunity to see either of their parents naked. Largely because of this lack of communication, children tend to hold a lot of false notions about sex. Not only does the sexual taboo result in their sexual ignorance, but it also conveys a certain attitude toward sexuality that strongly influences them when they are adults. In its milder forms, this attitude involves the feeling that sexuality is not to be openly admitted or expressed; it is a part of you that must be kept very private. In its more severe and debilitating forms, children develop the attitude that sex is dirty and sinful, something to be ashamed of. Exactly where you fit in along this range of attitudes depends to a large extent on your particular upbringing.

We learn as children that sexual feelings, even more than, say, anger, are not allowed free expression. Instead, we learn to fear our own sexuality and we work to keep it under strict control, expressing it only in certain ways and under certain circumstances. We learn that it can be expressed least of all in public, especially in the presence of children. It can be allowed somewhat freer expression in a bedroom late at night, when the children are asleep. Even there, however, people often find it impossible to escape the need for self-restraint. If they have children, they may be afraid that letting themselves go sexually will allow the children to realize what they're doing, and they believe this would be wrong. Sometimes there are no children; instead, it's a mother, another relation, or even the neighbors who are feared.

Even when they are completely alone, with no one around to worry about, many people are still left with their own negative sexual attitudes, which inhibit them. They fear that giving free expression to their sexual feelings will prove to be embarrassing, or worse. The most frequently expressed fear is that their partners would regard them as perverted, animalistic, promiscuous, or some such thing if they were to let themselves go. The result is that many, many people end up having sex in a quiet, self-conscious, self-restrained fashion. No wonder they don't enjoy it! The more severely negative are the attitudes we develop as children, the more afraid we usually are of letting go and the more inhibited we are during a sexual encounter. Our self-control may permit us to avoid feeling perverted, but at the price of sexual fulfillment.

People who complain that they don't enjoy sex or else feel that they seem to have little interest in it, in time can come to feel that there is something missing in *them*. What seems more true is that these people are either fearful about sex, unaccepting of their own sexuality, or both. Chapter 8 covers material for men who feel anxious about women, but in this section, we will focus on the second problem—denying your sexuality. This relates to the issue of *suppression* and the problems that a negative sexual attitude can create.

Persons whose upbringings led them to develop particularly strong negative (unaccepting) attitudes toward sex can fall into a habit, beginning at an early age, of suppressing and feeling ashamed of any sexual feelings. Suppression is a form of self-restraint. It is one way that people deal with the guilt and shame they may have about normal sexual thoughts, feelings, and urges. Suppressing sexual feelings throws a heavy blanket over them just as soon as they become recognizable for what they are. It does not seem possible for men to avoid sexual feelings completely (perhaps due to biological factors), but because they are so uncomfortable about these feelings, some men prefer to try to ignore or avoid them as much as possible rather than accepting them. The job these men do of covering up their own sexuality, especially from other people, can be very effective. No one looking at or talking to one of these men would ever suspect that he had sexual desires. Only he knows and feels guilty about them.

It is easy to see where consistently suppressing sexuality over a period of years can lead. After a while these people may conclude that they don't really have many sexual feelings left. Usually adults worry about sex when they or their partners feel that there is something missing from their relationship. They would like to feel more sexual desire and more comfort about sexuality, but find to their dismay that they are not very passionate and do not feel comfortable in bed.

The most difficult thing to overcome may be your own fears about being sexual, of what could happen to you if you began to accept rather than reject your sexual self. Usually this boils down to a fear of promiscuity—a fantasy that a crack in the dam will bring forth an overwhelming flood of craving sexual lust. Most people have similar fears about other aspects of themselves that they suppress, and it is to be expected. For example, people who suppress anger (because they learn as children that anger is unacceptable) have fears about what they would do if they became angry. Although such fears are expressed often, I have never yet met someone who turned into a raving killer simply because he or she expressed, rather than suppressed, anger, nor have I seen a person lose all self-control and be overcome by sexual lust, or end up turning into a sexual monster, as a result of trying to be less sexually inhibited. Instead, people seem very capable of letting themselves gradually become more sexual, while still setting limits on what they feel comfortable doing.

When you start letting yourself be sexual, you may experience desires that go against the grain of your moral values. You may begin, for instance, to have sexual "daydreams" or "nightdreams." If you are in a relationship, these fantasies will almost certainly involve persons other than your partner, at least some of the time. They may also include sexual acts you have never tried and even some that you might usually find offensive. You may experience homosexual fantasies, a strong interest in pornography, or compelling urges to look at women's bodies. Such reactions indicate that you are opening the doors of your sexuality, and they should not be taken to mean that you are losing all control over yourself. Again, this phenomenon is not unique to sex. Persons who deny themselves anything over a long period of time are likely to experience an urge to "gorge themselves" once they try it and find that they like it. For the overwhelming majority of people, this phase of the change process passes after a while. In an area as important as sexuality, in which feelings may be severely suppressed, this growth process may take a year or more.

If you are in a relationship, your new sexuality may catch your partner by surprise and throw the relationship temporarily off balance. After all, your sexual relationship has developed with you being one way—nonsexual or inhibited. Patterns have evolved based on this former sexual self that were familiar to both of you. By now your partner may be used to being the "sexy" one in the relationship and she may not entirely enjoy having this role taken away from her if you, too, start to become sexy. Also, although lack of sexuality may be a problem now, one reason for your partner's original attraction to you may have had to do with the fact that you did not come on as very sexual. Sometimes women feel uncomfortable around men who have a strong interest in sex, fearing perhaps that they may be too demanding, unfaithful, or both. As much as your partner may want it, your new-found sexuality may upset her by arousing whatever anxieties she may have about sexy men. It would be helpful if you could discuss these possibilities with her as you begin to change. You can assure her that because you are becoming sexier does not mean she is any less sexy and that you will not turn into a demanding, insatiable lecher.

On the other hand, your changing sexuality will mean that you both are going to do some adapting, and there may well be some risks involved (for instance, you may become interested in other women). Only you can decide whether the potential benefits are worth the risks. Since you are both involved, and since these sorts of things are always more difficult to deal with separately and in silence, approach them openly and together. You both stand to benefit from these changes, but at the same time you both stand to be affected by the risks that come with changing. You would be wise not to approach these issues with your eyes closed and your mouths shut.

In some ways you may already have experienced yourself becoming more sexual as a result of the exercises in the previous chapters. Think about this. In what ways are you different now, sexually? How do you feel about these changes? How does your partner feel about them? How has she changed? You may experience some anxiety now and again as a part of the change process. It would be useful if you could nail down the source of this tension. Is it because you still feel twinges of guilt, embarrassment, or shame about being sexual? How much of your anxiety has to do with fears about where all this will lead? Have you talked about these fears with each other?

APPEARANCES

One characteristic that is frequently typical of people who do not get much pleasure from their sexual relationship is that they are modest and self-controlled. A difficulty in letting go sexually, in other words, is often just one reflection of a broader trait of self-restraint. In their day-to-day lives, these people tend to be overly concerned with appearances, with the impression they give to others. Therefore, they spend a lot of time being self-conscious about what they say, what they do, how they look, and so forth. At the same time, the sexual image they present tends to be extremely downplayed. For instance, they seldom curse or tell dirty jokes; they would be embarrassed if they were "caught" looking at a woman in a sexual way; and they tend to avoid even the most normal sorts of flirtations. In their physical appearance they are careful not to give the impression of being particularly sexual; in fact, they often go to the opposite extreme and make themselves appear nonsexual.

Because a person is self-conscious and works hard to appear nonsexual to others does not mean that he or she has no sexual interests. Nothing could be further from the truth. These people do have sexual interests; they are simply hidden from view. Similarly, because a person does not express a strong interest in having sex with his or her partner does not mean that he or she has no sexual outlets. There are, besides sexual encounters, many ways to achieve sexual expression, including masturbation, dreams, and so on. People who are excessively inhibited often enjoy solitary sex more (they feel less self-conscious, more relaxed) than sex with a partner. Unfortunately, these people usually feel guilty about their private sexual activities and this attitude dampens their enjoyment of whatever means of sexual expression they do allow themselves.

Sexual self-consciousness and inhibition in adulthood seem to be very clearly a reflection of a person's experiences as a child and adolescent. People who are sexually self-restrained often have had either upbringings in which sexuality was stifled, or especially bad experiences (for example, rape), or both. Through observing parent's behavior children may learn that expressing sexual feelings, acting in a sexual way toward another person, even dressing in a manner that conveys sexuality are unacceptable in day-to-day living. Parents can also, through words and actions, cause children to feel that sex is dirty, disgusting, or wrong. Finally, religious dogmas often include strong sexual taboos and can create in children the impression that sex is sinful and, therefore, a part of themselves they should be ashamed of.

Regardless of the specific causes, men (and women) who are very sexually inhibited can almost always trace at least some of the roots of their sexual discomfort to childhood. For those who can't, the cause of their inhibition may not lie in parents or religion, but rather in some especially frightening sexual experiences. Boys who have experienced homosexual rape, who have suffered a venereal disease, or who have had the experience of being caught, for instance, in the act of masturbating or having sex with a girl and who were then punished or made to feel humiliated for this, can develop negative or nervous attitudes toward sex as adults. Because of their bad experiences they, too, may have a desire to hide their sexuality and limit its expression to "safe" circumstances (for example, masturbation).

Overcoming sexual inhibitions is a process in which a person gradually learns to let him- or herself be more sexual. It is good to approach this task in a gradual manner, since slow change generally seems easier to adapt to than rapid change. As a person becomes more sexual, he or she will have to cope with changes in other's reactions, as well as his or her own feelings. Make no mistake about it: if you have been sexually inhibited and modest, others will react to you differently as you begin to show the sexuality you have kept hidden. In all probability you will also have to deal with feelings of discomfort that come from feeling guilty or ashamed about sex. You will need to push yourself to do this, and you are probably better off doing it a little at a time.

The exercises in this chapter can guide you, but once more it will be up to you to do the actual work. If you are in a relationship, it can be a great help to discuss your feelings about, and reactions to, your changes with your partner and have her support and encouragement. Discussing it with a close friend or two, and having their support as well, can also be extremely helpful.

Exercise 4.1: Changing Your Appearance

Give some thought to your physical appearance and the ways you might change it in order to appear more sexual. Make *one* small change in your appearance each month for six months. Each time, make a change that will, in your opinion, cause you to look and feel a bit more sexy than you have in the past. The changes needn't be dramatic, but they should be noticeable, at least to people you are close to.

In looking for areas to change, consider the following list. Try not to make all of your changes in one area; spread them out a bit.

- Hair (length, style)
- Facial hair (beard, moustache)
- Glasses (style, color)
- Teeth
- Jewelry (bracelets, necklaces)

- Cologne
- Shirts
- Sweaters
- Slacks
- Belts
- Shoes
- Socks
- Coats and jackets

Remember that your changes are likely to arouse some discomfort in you and cause others to react to you in ways that make you feel uncomfortable. As is the case with all the other changes we have discussed, getting started is the hardest part. Your initial feelings of anxiety and guilt may make it difficult for you to begin making changes. At this point you will need to push yourself, and at this critical point the encouragement and support of others can be most helpful.

In considering what sorts of changes to make in your appearance, you may want to spend some time browsing through men's magazines and clothing stores. It can also be useful and fun to discuss your ideas with friends, or your partner, to get their opinion on what would suit you best. After you have done this, take some time to list in the spaces below the specific changes you plan to make in the forthcoming six months.

- Month 1 _____

- Month 2 _____

- Month 3 _____

- Month 4 _____

- Month 5 _____

- Month 6 _____

If you move one step at a time, in six months your appearance should be noticeably different. Moreover, by taking a gradual approach, your changes will be easier to cope with than they might be if you made many changes at once. After your six months are over, you can, of course, continue to make changes, but before you do, try to remember to read through this exercise again and answer the following questions for yourself.

List in the spaces below the specific changes in your appearance that you have made in the last six months.

_____

_____

_____

_____

_____

_____

In the space below, list any additional changes you plan to make in the forthcoming months.

_____

_____

_____

What, if any, sorts of reactions have you gotten from other people, including your partner, in response to the changes in your sexual appearance? How do you personally feel at this point about the changes you've made?

ENJOYING YOURSELF

Men and women alike are capable of enjoying themselves sexually, for example, by stimulating themselves to the point of orgasm. This sort of self-indulgence, however, has traditionally been discouraged—especially for women, but for men, too—while other forms of self-indulgence have not. For some reason it was thought that giving people permission to masturbate would result in their becoming too sexual, or that it would lead to less interest in having sex with a partner. Then, too, people once thought that masturbation was physically harmful and that in men it could lead to infertility. Apparently people believed that a man had only a fixed amount of sperm in his body, and that once it was used up there would be no more.

There is absolutely no evidence to support the idea that masturbating turns anyone into a sex fiend, or that it leads to infertility. We know now that a man's testes continue to produce sperm throughout his life, and if sperm is not ejaculated within a couple of days after reaching maturity, it disintegrates and is reabsorbed into the body. And contrary to the notion that masturbation is physically harmful is evidence to suggest that a total abstinence of any sexual outlet for a prolonged period of time can lead to prostate problems, loss of sexual interest, and erection difficulties in men, and to vaginal congestion and even shrinking of the vagina in women. In men, a lack of masturbation can also contribute to a tendency to ejaculate quickly.

Both men and women report that the orgasms they experience when they masturbate feel different from the ones they experience during sex with a partner, whether or not that sex involves intercourse. Some men say that the internal contractions accompanying orgasm feel more intense during masturbation or manual stimulation by a partner than they do during intercourse, but that they lack the pleasant feeling of vaginal containment and pressure that intercourse provides. Other men feel that their orgasms during intercourse are the most intense they can experience. Women, too, often state that the orgasms they give themselves feel different from the ones they have with a partner.

There is, then, a general consensus that the two kinds of orgasm feel different. Those who then go on to say that this difference will result in people becoming less interested in sex with a partner, and prefer masturbation instead, make two mistakes. First, they assume that masturbation orgasms feel better than partner orgasms. Second, they reduce sex to a purely physical, and specifically a genital, experience. But lovemaking is much more than genital pleasure. It is a way of getting close to another person, of giving, sharing, and communicating love. If it were not all these things, people would have given it up long ago, with or without permission. The act of making love with a partner is filled with meaning and emotion for both lovers. These factors are at least as important as the genital and other physical sensations that lovemaking gives us, and this is why people do it, want it, and like it, and why they feel so badly if their sexual relationships deteriorate.

Just as people will continue to engage in lovemaking, they will continue to masturbate, as is their natural right, for this is what they sometimes want and enjoy. To argue that it is wrong to want to masturbate so long as there is a willing partner available is only a little better than prohibiting it altogether. We all exist as individuals, just as much as we exist as part of a relationship. If we tie all of our needs, sexual or otherwise, into a relationship by saying that we *must* fill those needs through another person whenever possible, we set up an arbitrary, artificial barrier between ourselves and our needs. When we do that, we are saying that it is wrong to care for or enjoy ourselves. This is absurd. If you enjoy laughing, you might like it when your partner makes a joke, but you might also like to make yourself laugh sometimes, for instance, by thinking of a funny joke or situation. How would you feel if you were told that it was wrong to make yourself laugh or that it was right only if your partner wasn't there to tell you a joke? You would probably think this was ridiculous and would feel restricted and angry. It *would* be a ridiculous rule and you wouldn't obey it. The same thing applies to masturbation.

Masturbation is one way of enjoying yourself sexually. If you have had a typical sort of upbringing, you probably do masturbate and enjoy it, but you still would feel a little uncomfortable admitting the fact or talking to your partner about it.

Right now we will reevaluate your attitudes toward masturbation. Try to focus on its positive aspects and make a concentrated effort to challenge, in your own mind, the reasoning behind the old taboo about giving yourself pleasure.

Exercise 4.2: Pleasuring Yourself

This exercise will require about forty-five minutes of uninterrupted privacy. You will also need a bottle of baby oil, body lotion, or hand lotion, and you may want to keep a towel handy.

> Begin by taking a leisurely bath or shower. Take your time, and let the warmth of the water relax your muscles. Then go to your bedroom and lie down naked on your bed. Squeeze a bit of lotion on your hand and rub it in very well on both hands. If they get dry, apply a little more. Notice how smooth your skin feels when it is oiled. Now, stroke the back of one hand using the finger tips of the other. Focus your attention on the feelings in the hand that is being stroked. Switch, and stroke the other hand, again concentrating on how it feels to be stroked on your hand.

> Squeeze more lotion into your palm, rub the palms together to warm the lotion, and then spread it on your forearms. First, rub it in good, using long up-and-down strokes. Then touch yourself gently, caringly, affectionately. Use your finger tips to notice how your skin feels when it is oiled. Then shift your focus of attention and notice how your forearms feel when they are stroked in a gentle, caring manner.

> Apply lotion to your upper arms next. Follow the same procedure: rub the oil or lotion between your palms to warm it up, then apply it to your upper arms and rub it in a bit; shift from a firm touch to a gentle one, and notice, first, how your skin feels and, second, how it feels when it is stroked. Use this procedure to explore all the parts of your body.

> Apply the oil or lotion to your chest, making sure that, as always,

you first warm it up by rubbing it in your palms. Use both hands to rub it on your chest. Use your fingers to experience the way your chest feels when it is oiled. Then shift your attention and concentrate on how your chest feels when you stroke it. Try to stroke yourself with care and affection. Now, squeeze a bit more lotion onto your finger tips and begin rubbing it into your nipples. Stroke them gently and concentrate on how this feels. You may want to try out a sexual fantasy at this point, for example, imagining that it is a woman who is stroking you. Let yourself get into such a fantasy for a minute or two while you continue to stroke your chest and nipples. Let yourself feel sexually aroused if you like, but don't as yet begin touching your genitals.

Apply oil or lotion to your stomach next, rubbing it in firmly, then stroking yourself gently. Warm some more oil and apply it to your thighs. Stroke your thighs gently, on the outsides and on the insides. If you like, experiment again with having a sexual fantasy as you do so.

Next, do your calves, ankles, and feet. Don't skip over these parts of you (especially your feet) too quickly. As you apply lotion to your feet, use a light touch and continue with your sexual fantasy, imagining that it is a woman who is touching you. Run your fingers between your toes—does that feel good?

Now rub oil into your palms, roll over, and begin rubbing it into your buttocks. Then stroke your cheeks lightly and pay attention to how that feels. Imagine for a moment that it is a woman who is stroking you there, and stroke yourself the way you would want her to.

Roll over onto your back again and rub some more oil into your palms. Take your penis into your hands and begin to stroke it lightly. Notice the way the skin of your penis feels. Close your eyes and imagine that a woman whom you find sexually attractive is in bed with you and that she wants to stroke your body and genitals. She wants to please you as much as possible, in any way that you want. Begin touching your genitals in ways that you would like her to. Imagine that your hands are her hands. Stroke your penis, your scrotum, and your nipples, but touch yourself in other places as well. Make love to yourself in the way *you would like her to. Stimulate yourself to erection and then further. Do the sorts of things to yourself with your hands that you would want your lover to do. Imagine her doing these things to you. Stroke your penis harder. Imagine your lover's hands, holding you, stroking you, harder and harder. Stroke harder and faster until you reach orgasm. As you climax, imagine your lover's hands holding you tightly.*

How did that feel? Was it pleasant? If not, give some thought to why it might not have been an enjoyable experience for you. Did you feel guilty—that you were doing something dirty or sinful? If so, try to challenge the kind of thinking that says it is harmful or wrong to enjoy yourself. Trace back the origins of your superstitions about masturbation and put them on trial in your own mind. Defend your—and everyone's—right to give ourselves sexual pleasure.

If you suffer from strong feelings of guilt about sex, you may have to go through this mental exercise—challenging your inhibitions—many times before you begin to feel more comfortable pleasuring yourself. It will also be important that you continue to allow yourself to masturbate at least once a week, preferably more often. Push yourself to do this if it feels uncomfortable. Experiment with different sorts of sexual fantasies. Continue to use body oil or lotion as a regular or occasional part of your pleasuring session. After a while you may find yourself becoming more comfortable with the idea of self-pleasure and may make it a regular part of your life.

FANTASY

It is less of an embarrassment today than it once was for a person to admit to enjoying sexual fantasies. To say that you like to daydream about sex or to read sexy books now seems to be fairly acceptable. At the same time, it appears that it is just about as difficult for a man to admit to his partner that he likes to use fantasy occasionally during a sexual encounter as it is to admit that he sometimes prefers masturbation over intercourse. It is not something that is much discussed, but it is nevertheless true that most men of all ages fantasize, masturbate, and enjoy doing both.

Fantasizing during masturbation is very common. Most men imagine some sexual scene that helps to turn them on. The sexual fantasy provides them with psychic stimulation, while touching themselves gives them direct stimulation. Without the aid of the sexual fantasy (or some other form of psychic stimulation, such as pornographic pictures or stories), it would be more difficult for them to become aroused through direct stimulation alone to the point of climax. You might want to experiment with this for yourself. Begin masturbating without fantasizing (and without using any other aids, such as pictures or stories). If you are accustomed to using fantasy (or some other form of psychic stimulation) you will most likely find that your level of sexual arousal is not as high as it usually is. This is because you have deprived yourself of psychic stimulation by not fantasizing. When you let yourself fantasize again (or use some photos or a book), your level of sexual arousal will jump noticeably.

Many men and women feel comfortable fantasizing when they masturbate, but they feel somehow that it is (or would be) wrong to fantasize during a sexual encounter. They believe that fantasizing takes them away from the situation and that they owe it to their lover to stay in the situation. Or they believe that using fantasy means that you are not in love with your partner. Many people express such concerns about using sexual fantasies during a sexual encounter. If you should find yourself in a relationship in which you had to rely on fantasy as your *main* method of getting sexually aroused, you might need to reassess that relationship to discover why it is that other sources of arousal are closed off to you. On the other hand, if you simply use fantasy as *one of several* ways of getting turned on, you need not be concerned about it.

Another concern that people commonly express in regard to using sexual fantasies amounts to a fear that allowing yourself to indulge in a fantasy will mean that you will want to act it out. Frequently, people will fantasize about things they don't normally do. In fact, "wishful thinking" does seem to be an important function of fantasy. Just because you might enjoy thinking about something, however, does not mean that you would choose to do it even if you could. Having an urge, in other words, is different from acting on it. We all have urges; they are a normal part of living. Without this sort of outlet, life would certainly be more difficult to bear. At times when my work gets me down, I like to fantasize about being a farmer. Doing so makes me feel better—it helps me to forget my worries for a while. It does not mean, however, that I would really prefer being a farmer over what I do.

Aside from helping us feel better, fantasies often make us aware of the fact that we have many choices to make in life. Sometimes this can indeed be uncomfortable, but it, too, is inescapable. We do have to make choices, and it really is not possible to avoid doing so. I am aware of this when I enjoy fantasizing about having sex with different women I am attracted to. I choose not to try to act on such feelings, however, because I am more drawn to the intimacy of an exclusive sexual relationship than I am to the possibility of having many relationships. I have friends who are just the opposite; they do not prefer sexual exclusivity in reality, but they fantasize about it at times. They, too, must choose, and their fantasies reflect this.

Rather than trying to avoid temptation and the choices it forces upon you, accept this as a natural part of living. Permitting yourself to consider alternatives, and then choosing your preferred course of action, may be uncomfortable at times, but it also leads to a sense of personal strength. In sex, allow yourself to indulge in fantasies that turn you on and consider this a healthy, not unhealthy, behavior. If and when you ever find yourself in a position of being unable to decide what you want, a friend or counselor may be a good person to consult at that time. That would not mean that you were crazy or weak—only human.

Sexual fantasies tend to be private things, and whether you choose to share with your partner the fact that you fantasize, or what you like to fantasize about, is entirely up to you. A great many men expect that their partners would be offended if they were to acknowledge the use of sexual fantasies during a sexual encounter, much less disclose the contents of these fantasies. Actually, in my experience as a sex therapist, I have found that few women are really as put off by the idea as men seem to think. Women, of course, often fantasize, and sharing this part of their sexuality with one another more often than not seems to move a couple closer together.

Using sexual fantasies during a sexual encounter, like engaging in different sexual activities, is doing something that you like and adds to your sexual arousal and sense of satisfaction. In this case it is a form of psychic stimulation that you are using for your own benefit. Rather than being something that will replace other forms of stimulation, fantasy can be used, in addition to direct stimulation and other kinds of psychic stimulation, to enhance your sexual arousal. As opposed to relying solely on any one source of sexual stimulation, there is a great advantage to be had from using a "shuttling" technique: shifting your focus of attention from once source of stimulation to another. You may, for instance, move your attention from your partner's reactions or the way she looks (psychic stimulation), to your own physical sensation as your partner touches you (direct stimulation), to a sexual fantasy (psychic stimulation), and then back to your partner again. The result is that sexual arousal increases through the use of all of these channels of stimulation, and the sense of sexual fulfillment you can derive from the encounter is potentially that much greater.

Exercise 4.3: Developing Sexual Fantasy

If you are a person who does not fantasize very much about sex, but would like to experiment with this source of sexual arousal, you will do best to approach fantasizing as a skill that you can develop with practice. Begin by using the Sexual Fantasy Record below to record *any and all sexual thoughts* you might have each day for one week. Include all of the following on your record:

1. Sexual thoughts you might have about women you know or meet.
2. Any incidents you might read about, hear about, see, or make up for yourself that seem to arouse you sexually, even a little bit.
3. Fantasies you might have while masturbating.
4. Any exciting sexual night dreams you can recall.

As an additional aid for stimulating your fantasy life, you might want to look through some men's magazines (many have columns devoted to sexual fantasies; the pictures and stories in them may suggest fantasies) or read some sexy novels.

SEXUAL FANTASY RECORD

For each day of the week, make a note of all your sexual thoughts and fantasies

MONDAY

TUESDAY

WEDNESDAY

THURSDAY

FRIDAY

SATURDAY

SUNDAY

At first your Fantasy Record may contain few entries, but you should notice a slow, steady increase over time. If progress after one week seems especially slow, repeat this step for a second week. At the end of that time, go through your record(s) and make a mental note of the contents. Which sorts of fantasies seem to turn you on the most?

As a second step, take a few blank sheets of paper, sit in a private place, and spend one-half hour or more writing a description of the *most sexually exciting scene you can imagine*. You can destroy these sheets afterward if you like, but perhaps you should keep them in a safe place. Repeat this part of the exercise again a few days later, this time trying to write out a sexually stimulating fantasy that is different from the first one you wrote.

As a third step in learning to use fantasies, try to make up a sexual fantasy that appeals to you, and use it, a little at a time, while you masturbate. You may want to use photos from a magazine, part of a story you read, material from your Sexual Fantasy Record, or the sexual fantasies you created. See if, when used in this way, the fantasy can add to your level of arousal. Experiment with different fantasies to see which are the most arousing for you. Continue with this step until you feel comfortable using fantasy while you masturbate.

Once you are successfully fantasizing during masturbation, begin experimenting with using fantasy during a sexual encounter as an additional means of getting excited. Again, you would do best to try it out briefly at first, at a point when you're already feeling aroused. If you begin to feel uncomfortable, it may be because you feel guilty about fantasizing in this situation, but it may also be due to the fact that it is something new and takes some getting used to. Avoid any tendency to rely exclusively on your sexual fantasy to become aroused; use it instead as one of several sources of arousal. Shuttle your focus of attention, from the fantasy, to your partner, to your own body sensations. Give yourself time to develop the skill of using sexual fantasy, as well as the skill of shuttling.

FACILITATING SEXUAL EXPRESSION

Part of the general attitude of self-restraint that stands in the way of sexual fulfillment for many men involves controlling the expression of sexual feelings and reactions during lovemaking. Men who complain of feeling unfulfilled reveal that they feel as though they make love stiffly and that they seem to be stuck in one routine. They tend to be self-conscious all or most of the time and are often aware that they purposely hold back. The idea of letting go—of making noise, moving around, or trying something on the spur of the moment—scares them. Their fear seems to be one of losing control: something bad (or at least embarrassing) would happen if they let themselves go. This type of suppression is another manifestation of negative sexual attitudes. In the exercises in this section you will be asked to experiment with letting go a bit, specifically by moving around and expressing, rather than holding back, your sexual feelings and reactions.

Exercise 4.4: Letting Go Alone

Find a time when you can be alone in your house or apartment and can have a good half-hour or more of total privacy.

Make yourself comfortable in your bed and begin to masturbate. Use fantasies, a men's magazine, or whatever turns you on. Start off by touching yourself in places other than your genitals. As you begin to experience some sexual arousal, begin at the same time to move your pelvis. Move it rhythmically from side to side, up and down. Move around slowly at first, then a little faster. Next, try moving your legs a little. Rub them together. Then move the trunk of your body and your abdomen. If your breathing seems tight, purposely try to make it deeper, heavier. As you start feeling more comfortable moving around a little, begin to moan, groan, or say something to express the feelings and reactions you are experiencing. Do this out loud. Try out different ways of expressing your feelings. If you like, start out with moaning and then experiment with making different sounds. Say things like: "Oh! Wow!" At first you can make your sounds soft and low, but let yourself gradually get a bit louder. Similarly, make small body movements at first, but try letting yourself make bigger movements as time goes on.

Now begin stimulating your genitals. Take your penis in your hand and stroke it. Stroke your scrotum as well, using your other hand. Continue to let yourself move around. Try to establish a coordinated rhythm between your strokes and pelvic movements. At the same time, work on expressing, out loud, your reactions, rather than holding them back. Let yourself move more and more and express yourself louder and louder. See how good it can feel to let yourself go. Continue stroking yourself, harder and harder, faster and faster. Let your breathing get heavier and heavier, louder and louder. As you reach orgasm, let yourself make your loudest sound yet—an uncensored expression of pleasure!

When you reach orgasm during these sessions, try to avoid any tendency to use a tissue or some such thing to come into. If you are afraid of making a mess, put a towel under you. Better still, forget about making a mess. Just let yourself come without holding back or worrying about being "clean" about it.

What was that like for you? Did you feel awkward at first? That is to be expected if you are not used to moving around or giving voice to your feelings. Was the idea of moving around and making noise frightening or embarrassing to you? When you are used to holding back, the idea of letting go can arouse feelings of shame and/or anxiety. The shame would come from an attitude that sex is bad, dirty, or sinful. The anxiety would reflect a belief that sexual feelings should be feared—that they can take you over and turn you into a Mr. Hyde. Where do you think you might have gotten such attitudes? What are your beliefs now? Do you feel that sexual pleasure is sinful or debasing, or that something terrible will happen if you lose your self-control? Be honest with yourself. If you do tend to hold such beliefs, you must recognize that they contribute to your self-restraint and your self-consciousness. Learning to be less inhibited, freer, will then be a slower process for you. You will need to move at a pace that feels comfortable and safe. As you begin to feel less ashamed or embarrassed, and as you begin to see that you can let yourself go and not turn into a fiend, things will get easier. To reach this goal, you may need to repeat this exercise many times, perhaps twice a week.

Exercise 4.5: Letting Go with Your Partner

Usually people who feel sexually self-restrained and self-conscious are concerned about being able to let go when they are making love with a partner. However, since this is almost always more difficult than letting go when alone, Exercise 4.4 was included as a sort of intermediate step. This particular procedure of learning to do things alone, and then with a partner, has been found to be an effective way of changing sexual behavior.

Once you begin to feel more comfortable letting yourself go when you are alone, you can start experimenting with doing the same sorts of things when you are with a partner. You can expect to have to push yourself again, but having practiced by yourself should make it easier. You should also expect to feel at least a little embarrassed, or shy, at first. With persistence, however, as well as a positive response from your partner, this phase should quickly pass.

Before you begin to experiment with expressing your sexual feelings more in your sexual relationship, give some thought to any concerns you might have about doing so. Specifically, give some thought to your expectations about how your partner will react if you begin to do the same sorts of things with her that you did by yourself in Exercise 4.4. Do you think she would like or dislike it? Do you expect she would think less of you, in one way or another, as a result of your letting go? Chances are her impression of you *will* change: you will seem more sexual to her. Would this be okay with you?

You may want to try talking with your partner ahead of time about some of the issues and questions raised in the above paragraph. Your goal in this discussion should be to share as honestly as you can your potential concerns about letting go and to find out how your partner feels about it. You might also want to find out if she, too, feels sexually self-restrained and whether she would like to change.

When you feel ready to start experimenting with letting down your guard during sex, you would do best to proceed in the same fashion as you did in the previous exercise. That is, start off slowly and make your way gradually toward freer and freer expression. You may need to push yourself, but give yourself time and make progress at a reasonably comfortable pace. The following guidelines may be helpful.

If you haven't done so as yet, read the section on Sexual Communication in chapter 3 and work on developing the sorts of skills described there.

Try to arrange your sexual encounters so that your partner spends time doing things to you, as well as you doing things to her. During those times when she is pleasuring you, begin letting yourself express your reactions more by moving your body and making sounds in response to what she does.

Pay some attention to your breathing now and then. If it is tight, shallow, and constricted, let it become deeper, heavier. Let yourself pant, if that is what feels good, or release your feelings in big sighs. In short, don't stifle your breathing.

If you find yourself being self-conscious (as though you were standing back and watching the action like an observer), break this pattern by focusing your attention on something else—a sexual fantasy, your partner's responses, or the feelings in your own body.

Experiment with talking to each other during lovemaking. Tell your partner what feels good and ask her to tell you what feels good.

> *Try especially hard to get past your self-restraint as you reach orgasm. Let yourself moan, groan, or even shout if you want to. Try not to be afraid of showing your partner just how good you feel. Also, as in Exercise 4.4, don't let yourself get concerned with making a "mess" when you come, if that happens outside of your partner's vagina. Put some towels underneath you, if that would make you feel better, but don't try to ejaculate into something. Just let it happen, and focus your attention on the feelings, not on being self-conscious about neatness.*
>
> *Continue to share your feelings, between sexual encounters, with your partner about the changes you are making. Tell her any concerns you might have about becoming more sexually expressive and find out what her real feelings are about these changes.*

In contrast to their fears of being thought less of, men will generally find that their partners enjoy their increased sexual expressiveness. Most women find that a sexually responsive, as opposed to self-restrained, partner adds to their own level of sexual arousal and makes a sexual encounter more pleasurable. Your responsiveness, remember, will provide your partner with psychic stimulation. If you doubt this, consider how her responses to your lovemaking are a turn-on for you.

If it happens that both you and your partner tend to be sexually inhibited, you will need to help each other to become freer. If you tried working on this by yourself, your partner might react negatively out of her own feelings of shame or embarrassment, which will in turn discourage you. Working together to encourage each other to become more sexually expressive will reduce the stumbling blocks for each of you.

SEXUAL HISTORIES

One result of living in our culture, in which sex is such a taboo subject, is that people rarely have the opportunity to talk about their sexual experiences with others. In consequence, most of us end up feeling isolated, at least in terms of our sexual lives. Sharing experiences with someone who takes an understanding, sympathetic attitude is always a pleasant human activity. This is true regardless of what the particular experiences are. However, if they happen to be uncomfortable experiences, or ones that have never before been shared, the act of sharing can be an especially powerful event. If this sharing is two-way, it then becomes powerful for both people, drawing them closer and strengthening the bond between them.

Sharing experiences in an atmosphere of acceptance brings two people into contact with one another in a way that seems relatively rare. To achieve this goal, you need to learn how to listen, that is, to be ready to hear what someone else says and to accept it, without offering advice or placing judgment on what is said. This may not be easy for you to do. You may be tempted to judge others on the basis of their experiences; to say that they were good or bad because they had some experience. You may also be tempted to offer advice concerning, for example, what they "should" have done in some situation. If you take either of these attitudes, the chances are that the other person will feel a need to defend him- or herself and will not experience positive and intimate sharing with you.

One technique that is useful in helping to overcome judgmental attitudes is to try, as you listen, to place yourself in the other person's shoes. Another useful approach is to try to identify similar experiences that you yourself have had. If you do this, and refrain from casting judgment on the other person, you will maximize the chances that your sharing experiences will be good ones.

Think about your feelings about sharing things from your sexual past, as well as your present sexuality, that you have not before shared with your partner. Does the idea make you anxious? If so, what is your anxiety about? What sort of reaction are you afraid you might get in response, say, to talking about your early experiences with masturbation or sex play with girls? What sort of reaction would you fear getting in response to talking about your current masturbation practices or sexual fantasies? Do you think that the reactions you *might* get are the reactions your partner would *really* express? Would it be all right if your partner did get upset, if you felt that she would come around in a day or so?

How would you feel hearing your partner talk about topics such as those mentioned above? Do you think you could accept what she might say with a sympathetic attitude? What sorts of things that she might say would get you upset? Do you think you would get over being upset?

It would be a good idea if, before attempting the exercise in this section, you and your partner sit down together and talk, not about your sexual past, but about your concerns about sharing such information with each other. Talk about the sorts of reactions you fear getting in response to disclosing things and, if possible, which particular topics make you most nervous. Tell each other how you would like the other person to react to such an experience of sharing. Be as honest with each other as you can. If you think that something might get you upset, say so. If this discussion makes you feel more comfortable and ready to take the risk of sharing your sexual histories with each other, proceed with the following exercise.

Exercise 4.6: Sharing Your Sexual History

This exercise will take at least two hours, and probably longer. You may not be able to complete it in one sitting and may need to break it up into a series of sessions. You may also want to spread these sessions over a period of time, say a month or two. You will do best to take one section in the following outline at a time and take turns sharing information. Share as much as you feel you can, that is, be as open as you feel safe doing. If at any point you feel nervous about sharing something, talk to your partner about your anxiety before sharing the material. If you feel reassured that she or he is really interested and will be able to accept you even if what you are saying is upsetting, take the risk and be open.

SEXUAL HISTORY OUTLINE

Early Childhood

Share information with each other about each of the following:

- Your parents' socioeconomic, cultural, and religious background: what their upbringings, or roots, were like.
- Your parents' life-styles: the things they spend (or spent) their time doing, how they fill up their days and weeks.
- Your parents' personalities: brief descriptions of what sort of person each of them is (or was).
- Your parents' religious and moral attitudes.
- Your parents' attitudes toward play and leisure; what they like to do to relax and enjoy themselves and each other.
- Your memories of your parents' marital relationships: happy/unhappy, affectionate/unaffectionate, and so on.
- Any memories of thoughts or experiences you had as a child that had to do with your parents' sexual relationships.
- Your parents' attitude toward nudity in the home.
- Your parents' general attitudes about sex.
- Comments made to you by either of your parents concerning sex.
- Your recollections of any comments passed between your parents concerning sex.
- Your present thoughts about what sort of marriages and what kind of sexual relationships your parents have or may have had.
- What sorts of attitudes toward sex you developed as a child.
- Any bad (embarrassing, humiliating, frightening) sexual experiences you had as a child.
- Where, when, and how you first learned about the differences between boys and girls. What your reaction to this knowledge was.
- Any family crises you can remember.
- Any crises in your parents' marriages that you can remember.

Late Childhood and Adolescence

- Where, when, and from whom you first learned about the facts of life. What your reactions were to learning this.
- Any experiences you had concerning asking your parents about sex, or their telling you about it.

- Conversations about sex you had with your friends (note especially any incorrect information you may have believed).
- Your first experiences with masturbation: where you did it, how often you did it, how you felt about doing it.
- Any bad sexual experiences you may have had during this time in your life.

Men Only
- Your first wet dream or ejaculation: how you reacted, how your parents (if they found out) reacted.
- Your earliest sexual experience with a girl: how old you were, how old she was, what happened, how you each reacted.

Women Only
- Your first menstruation: how old you were, how you and your parents reacted.
- Your earliest sex play experiences with boys: how old you were, what you did, what, if anything, happened afterward, how you felt about it, during and after.

Adulthood
- Your early dating experiences: what sorts of girls (boys) you dated, your attitude about dating, how often you dated, how you felt about it.
- Your feelings about your own physical appearance and your sexual attractiveness.
- Your early experiences with kissing and petting: who, where, when, what your and their reactions were.
- Your first crush: who, when, their feelings about you, how it ended.
- Any embarrassing or frightening sexual experiences you have had as an adult.
- Your current attitudes about love.
- Your current attitudes about marriage.
- Any exceptionally good sexual experiences you have had as an adult.
- Your sexual night dreams and fantasies.
- Your current feelings about masturbation.
- Your reactions to pornography.

- Your feelings about what it would be like to be a very sexual person.
- Your feelings about what it would be like if your partner were a very sexual person.
- How you might like to be different than you are, sexually speaking.

The above is only a partial list of the sorts of things you might discuss during your time together. The outline is intended to provoke your memory and stir your current thinking. Feel free to pursue further any question that seems particularly important to you.

SUMMARY

This chapter is devoted to furthering your sexual development beyond the level presented in chapter 3. The exercises are designed to facilitate behavioral change in those people who are able to muster the necessary motivation to try them. Although most of these exercises can benefit you as an individual, the possibilities for personal growth are increased when two people work cooperatively to make changes they both see as desirable.

The sections in this chapter focus on areas that, if you develop your sexuality in each of them, will further facilitate change in your sexual relationship. They are all areas that tend to be more or less undeveloped in people who feel sexually dissatisfied and frustrated. Much of the excessive self-restraint and self-consciousness such people are burdened with reflects negative or fearful attitudes about being sexual. These attitudes in turn have their roots, for the most part, in an individual's specific upbringing and in the general sexual atmosphere that characterizes our culture. At this point, however, gnashing your teeth over society's shortcomings or feeling angry at your parents is not as likely to lead to positive change as is pushing yourself to try new things. If you are willing, and if you have the support of your partner, you have within you the power to change things for the better right now.

5 learning to relax

The two most frequent sexual complaints expressed by the men I have worked with professionally are a loss of sexual desire and difficulties in being able to relax during sex. To a large extent the material in chapters 2, 3, and 4 may be useful to men who have experienced a loss of sexual desire, as well as those who have never had a strong interest in sex. The second major sexual complaint—difficulty in relaxing—is covered in this and the following chapters. Because it is so useful, the *relaxation technique,* which is the subject of this chapter, will also be utilized in later chapters dealing with overcoming fears of women, erection difficulties, and so on.

Needless to say, there can be a great many different reasons why a man might find it difficult to relax or might feel sexually unfulfilled. What is responsible for one man's problem may not have much to do with another's. Despite this obvious fact, there may be some general causes of sexual dissatisfaction, circumstances that are shared by nearly all men and that may account for the fact that certain complaints, such as difficulty in relaxing, are so common. Two such general factors that seem particularly relevant are: the attitude that men are encouraged to take toward certain emotions within themselves, and the male sexual script, which gives the man all, or nearly all, of the responsibility for the content of a sexual encounter.

Taking responsibility for what happens during lovemaking forces a man to approach it self-consciously, as though it were a performance, something he can either "pass" or "fail" at. Whenever *any* situation, sexual or otherwise, is consistently approached in this manner, it tends to create a certain amount of nervous tension, or *performance anxiety*. In other words, whenever you invest yourself in an activity in such a way that it becomes a task, it is difficult not to be somewhat tense about it since you cannot help being concerned about how you will do. Just how tense you will feel depends upon several factors, including how well you think you ought to do, how important success at the particular task is to you, and your previous experiences with it. If you set your goals extremely high, you increase your chances of feeling tense (as well as failing). If success in this particular area is extremely important to you, you will again feel more tense than you would if it were less important. Finally, if you have had experiences in the past of not performing up to your expectations at the task, you will feel more tense than you would if you had more reason to believe you would do well.

These rules apply to sex as well as to any other task. If you expect that you must be a superlover, if sexual prowess is all-important to you, and/or if you have had disappointing experiences in the past (that is, not living up to your expectations), your sexual performance anxiety will be high. In contrast, to the extent that it is not so important that you be a superlover and that you have invested in things other than sex for feeling good about yourself, and the more you have been able to meet your expectations in the past, the lower your sexual performance anxiety will be.

One way to try to reduce sexual performance anxiety is to

develop some skill in relaxing yourself. The technique described in this chapter is designed to do that. By itself, however, learning to relax may not be enough. What is equally important to overcoming performance anxiety is to make sex into less of a performance. As a man, this means giving some of the responsibility for the quality of your sexual relationship to your partner. Giving more responsibility means that you will lose some responsibility. As desirable as this may be, in practice men frequently feel uncomfortable, anxious, and even threatened when they give up some responsibility and control. They may perceive their partner as being overly aggressive, or they may fear that she will become "oversexed" and will make demands that they will not be able to meet. These initial reactions are to be expected, and they will pass in time. The key to getting through them is new experience, seeing for yourself that shared responsibility will not lead to disaster.

Women can also have negative reactions to changes in their sexual relationships with their partners. For them the idea of having more responsibility and control may appeal on an intellectual level, but on an emotional level they might not be so comfortable with it. Women frequently say that they feel awkward, for instance, taking the initiative in sex, and some report that they find it difficult to get sexually aroused *unless* their partner is in control. They may begin to experience performance anxiety themselves, being self-conscious and worrying if they are doing well. Getting past these sorts of difficulties will take time, and it may be necessary to make changes in steps rather than all at once. Women will find that they need to push themselves to try new things just as much as men do; the section on Sexual Communication in chapter 3 can be helpful in this regard. Also helpful will be your ability to talk to each other, in between sexual encounters, about your reactions to changing. If you can support and encourage each other, your chances of success will be that much greater.

For those people who feel that difficulties in relaxing are interfering with their sexual enjoyment, this chapter and the next are especially important. You will learn to pay attention to your own body, to develop some sensitivity in detecting tension. You will learn a specific technique to relax yourself when you discover that you are tense. Finally, you will be asked to make a start in learning to build body awareness and to apply the relaxation technique toward day-to-day life. With this foundation, the exercises in chapter 6 will help you to deal specifically with the problem of tension in sexual situations.

TENSION AND RELAXATION

Often when I ask a man how he is feeling, the response is a look of surprise. It is also common for the man to look confused, shrug his shoulders, and say, "I don't know." Or he may respond with something noncommital, like "all right" or "okay." A great many men—probably the vast majority—seem distinctly uncomfortable being asked about their feelings, and they prefer to move on to some other topic of conversation. This is not difficult to understand if you view it from the perspective of the way in which men are raised. Through childhood, and especially during adolescence, boys pick up a set of expectations concerning how they should act as men. At the same time, girls are learning what will be expected of them as women. Men are expected to act in certain ways, women in other ways, in all sorts of situations. For instance, men are expected to be brave, competitive, independent, and persevering. As we strive to become men, each of us usually tries to live up to these expectations as best we can. As admirable as we might consider such qualities to be, the pursuit of such traits as ideals has its drawbacks. One of the most serious drawbacks is that the role men are expected to fill, and which they more often than not try to live up to, requires them to learn to suppress a lot of feelings, especially fear or anxiety, loneliness or discouragement. Sometimes, it seems, men can even learn to suppress affection and love, becoming capable of doing very hurtful things to others.

Men are not naturally unfeeling. They are, however, consistently encouraged from an early age to deny or control their feelings, for example, by being told that they should not let feelings "get in the way" of their competitive pursuits. From expressions like "keep a stiff upper lip" and the like, men come to be ashamed of any tendency to give in to tender emotions. No wonder that by the time they are thirty years old, it is so difficult for men to cry or to admit to feeling weak, afraid, lonely, or discouraged. It is an important personal decision as to whether you as an individual man want to accept or reject the role you have been raised to fulfill. If you do want to change, you stand to profit. But you should not expect the change process to be an easy one. In trying to change your role as a man, you will be going against old habits and also against the grain of our culture. You will not be alone among men, but neither will you be in the majority.

We are concerned here mainly with just one aspect of the larger male sex role. That aspect has to do with the issue of nervous tension, or anxiety, and your ability to detect it and deal with it. It is a concern because one of the feelings that men usually try to suppress—to put out of their minds—is anxiety. That men should learn to suppress anxiety makes sense, because getting in touch with such feelings makes it more difficult to be competitive, brave, persevering, and so forth. What you don't know, in other words, can't hurt you. As a result of years of effort aimed at suppressing nervous tension, most men get to a point where they are no longer aware of it when they are feeling tense. Since tension is a major cause of sexual, as well as other physical, difficulties, this means that men who are experiencing such problems are at a disadvantage in dealing with them; that is, what they don't know does hurt them.

Learning to perceive your own level of tension is the aim of this and the next exercise. If you are like most men, you could look scared to death, but if someone asked you if you were tense, you would think they were crazy to suspect such a thing. Some of the times you would know very well that you were tense and would just not want to admit it. But many times you would be responding truthfully in this situation; you really would not realize you were anxious. Developing an ability to perceive your own level of tension is, therefore, a skill that you need to develop. It is a skill you most certainly can learn, but which, like learning any other skill, requires practice, patience, and motivation. You can start learning to identify tension by exaggerating it. By doing so, the difference between tension and relaxation will gradually become clearer. At the same time, you will be learning a technique that can help you to relax yourself at times when you do feel tense.

Exercise 5.1: Tension Versus Relaxation

To be aware that you are either tense or relaxed is actually a simple process, but it requires practice at first if you are not used to doing it. Briefly, what it involves is learning to pay attention to the level of tension in the muscles of the various parts of your body (back, neck, stomach, and so on) and to your breathing, and to notice differences in these things in different situations. Chances are that you are not very much aware of the different tension levels in your body right now or of the way you happen to be breathing. As a beginning, therefore, lie down on your back someplace, preferably a hard surface like a bare floor or carpet, with this book in your hand. Do this right now, before you read on.

Now that you are lying flat, hold this book above and in front of you. Focus your attention on the muscles in the hand and arm that are holding up the book. Pay close attention to how these muscles feel at this moment.

Slowly put your arm and the book down on the floor beside you, and as you are doing so, keep your attention focused on the muscles in your hand and arm. Is there a difference *in the level of tension in your muscles under these two circumstances (book and arm up versus book and arm down)? Are you aware of the* change *in the level of tension in your arm as you let it down?*

Repeat the above procedure. Lift the book up and hold it in front of you; focus on the feelings in the muscles of your hand and arm; slowly let the book down; focus on the feelings again.

Chances are that you did perceive a difference—there was more tension in your arm when it was holding the book up than when it was down at your side. You may also have noticed the tension level changing as you lowered your arm and let it rest against the floor.

Shift your attention now to each of the following parts of your body, one at a time, but not too fast: face, neck, and shoulders; arms and hands; chest, back, and stomach; genitals, buttocks, legs, and feet. Be sure to focus on each part for a moment before moving on.

Did you notice, in checking out the different parts of your body, that the muscles in some places felt more tense than those in other parts? If not, look again—it is almost certain that there are some differences you can detect. Which areas seem more tense; which seem more relaxed?

This exercise is designed to introduce you to the idea of paying attention to your body and noticing the different levels of tension in it. Anxiety, or nervous tension, is not something that exists only in a person's mind. If you are feeling tense, your body will reflect this fact. Because men tend to try to put thoughts of anxiety out of their minds, a good way for them to learn to detect tension in themselves is for them to begin paying attention to their bodies.

THE RELAXATION TECHNIQUE

The technique used in the previous section to help you experience the difference between tension and relaxation can be extended into a method you can use to relax yourself when you are feeling tense.

Exercise 5.2: Learning the Relaxation Technique

Find a comfortable chair to sit in. If you don't have a comfortable chair, lie down on a rug, a couch, or your bed. Read through this entire exercise carefully and completely before beginning, then take the instructions with you to refer to as you go along. If you have a tape recorder, you may wish to record the instructions and play them back. If you do this, be sure to speak slowly and clearly. Also, stop for as long as the instructions request each time you come to the word "pause" in parenthesis, for example (**Pause fifteen seconds**); leave the recorder running. After the pause, continue reading the instructions into your recorder, slowly and clearly. Although it may take you some time to make a relaxation tape, it will probably be worth it.

> *Begin by lying (or sitting) down. Take a deep breath, then another. Each time you breathe, try to inhale and exhale deeply. Breathe by letting your stomach move in and out. Practice this method of breathing for a minute or so before going on.*
>
> *(**Pause one minute.**)*
>
> *Clench your left hand. Make it into a tight fist. Clench it as tightly as you can and hold it that way. Focus your attention on the feelings of tension in the muscles of your hand and arm, your fingers and wrist. Do you feel it? Now, say the word RELAX out loud and at the same time let your hand relax. Pay attention to the feelings of your muscles relaxing.*
>
> *(**Pause ten seconds.**)*
>
> *Repeat the above sequence: Tense your left hand tightly and hold the tension; focus on the way it feels; say the word RELAX out loud and let the tension go. Focus on the feelings of relaxation.*
>
> *(**Pause ten seconds.**)*
>
> *Now make your right hand into a fist. Clench the muscles tightly and hold them that way. Notice this feeling of tension and what it is like. Say the word RELAX out loud, and as you do let your*

right hand relax. Note the way the muscles feel as tension leaves them. Notice also the way that relaxation feels and the difference between tension and relaxation.

(Pause ten seconds.)

Repeat the above procedure: tense your right hand; hold the tension and focus on it; say the word RELAX and let the tension go; focus on the feeling of relaxation.

(Pause ten seconds.)

Tense the muscles in both of your arms now. Make them very tense and hold that level of tension for a moment while you focus on the way it feels. Pay attention to how the tension feels, first in your right arm, then in your left arm. Say the word RELAX out loud and let your arms relax. Focus your attention on the feelings of tension draining away and on the way that relaxation feels afterward.

(Pause ten seconds.)

Repeat the above procedure: tense both arms; tense them hard and hold the tension; focus on the feelings; say the word RELAX and let the tension go; feel the tension draining away and the sensations of relaxation that follow.

(Pause ten seconds.)

Use this same procedure with the muscles in your jaw. Clench your jaw, tightly but not too tight. Hold that tension. Notice how it feels. Now, instead of saying the word RELAX, just think it. Think it very clearly, and as you do, allow your jaw to relax. Focus your attention on the feelings in your jaw muscles as the tension leaves them and then on how they feel when they are relaxed.

(Pause ten seconds.)

Repeat the tension and relaxation procedure with your jaw: clench your jaw and hold the tension, focusing on the feelings in the muscles; think the word RELAX and then let the tension go, focusing on the feelings of tension as they drain away and on the feelings of relaxation that follow.

(Pause ten seconds.)

Tense your neck and shoulders by hunching up. Hunch up tightly and hold the tension. Feel the tension in your shoulders and neck. Think the word RELAX and let the tension go. Notice the sensation of tension draining away. It almost seems to evaporate. Experience the sensation of relaxation in your neck and shoulders.

*(**Pause ten seconds.**)*

Repeat the tensing of your neck and shoulders: hunch up tightly and hold it, focusing on the way the muscles feel when they are all tense; think the word RELAX and let the tension go; focus on the sensation of tension leaving and the way the muscles feel afterward, when they have relaxed.

*(**Pause ten seconds.**)*

Now tense the muscles in your chest. Do this by taking in a deep breath and holding it. Keep on holding it and notice how it feels to be tense in your chest, to stop breathing. Now, think the word RELAX and let the tension go. Feel the tension leaving you. Exhale deeply and then breathe in deeply. Notice how it feels to breathe, deeply, easily, without tension. Tension and relaxation are very different, and by now this should be clearer and clearer.

*(**Pause ten seconds.**)*

Take in another deep breath and hold it. Tense the muscles in your chest. Hold the tension and your breath and focus on the way this feels. Think the word RELAX, exhale, and let the tension evaporate. Notice the way this feels. Inhale deeply and easily. See how good it is to breathe and how different it is from being all tensed up. Let yourself breathe deeply and easily for a minute. Breathe by letting your stomach move in and out.

*(**Pause one minute.**)*

You will notice that you are slowly working your way through your body. At each step along the way, you must tense your muscles, hold that tension, and notice how it feels by paying close attention to it. Then you say or think the word RELAX and at the same time let the tension go. Pay attention to the feelings of tension leaving, to the way that relaxation feels afterward, and to the difference between tension and relaxation. Follow this procedure now with your stomach. Tense the muscles in your stomach by drawing it in. Hold the tension. Experience it by paying attention to it. Think the word RELAX and let the tension drain from your stomach. Let it loose. Notice the feeling of tension draining off and then how it feels to be relaxed.

*(*Pause ten seconds.*)*

Tense your stomach again. Suck it in, hold the tension, and focus your attention on it. Think the word RELAX and let the tension go. Focus on the tension leaving and on the relaxation that follows. Notice the difference between tension and relaxation.

*(*Pause ten seconds.*)*

Tense up the muscles in your buttocks. Tense them tight by pulling them in, and hold that level of tension. Notice the way tension in that area feels. Think the word RELAX and at the same time let the muscles in your buttocks relax. Feel the tension leaving, and then experience the sensation of relaxation that follows.

*(*Pause ten seconds.*)*

Repeat the tensing and relaxing of your buttocks. Tense the muscles and hold them tense, focusing on the sensations of tension. Think the word RELAX and let the tension flow away. Just let it go. Feel it leaving you, and experience the sensation of relaxation.

*(*Pause ten seconds.*)*

Try now to tense the muscles in the pelvic region of your body. These muscles are located within your body, sort of behind and just above your genitals. When these muscles are tense (contracted), your penis may move a little. If you are not sure just which muscles are involved, imagine that you are urinating and want to stop the stream for a moment. The muscles you use to do this are the muscles you should tense up right now. Hold them at a moderate, not extreme, level of tension. Make them sufficiently tense, however, so that you can experience the tension when you focus your attention on it. Notice the way this particular form of tension feels. Now think the word RELAX and let these muscles relax. Let the tension go from your pelvis and focus on the way this feels. Now focus on the way that relaxation feels after all the tension is gone.

*(***Pause ten seconds.***)*

Tense your pelvic muscles again. Hold the tension and focus on it. Now think the word RELAX and let the tension go. Notice the feelings of relaxation.

*(***Pause ten seconds.***)*

The last muscle groups are those in your legs. Tense up the muscles in both of your legs right now. Make them very tense and hold that level of tension. Tense your thighs and lower legs. Notice the way tension in your legs feels. Think the word RELAX and let the tension go. Did you notice how it felt to let tension go? Note the way that relaxation feels.

*(***Pause ten seconds.***)*

Tense your legs once more. Hold the tension in them for a moment while you focus on the way they feel when they are all tight. Now think the word RELAX and let the tension go. Notice the change as it is taking place and the feeling of relaxation that follows.

It is strongly recommended that you practice Exercise 5.2 once a day, if possible, for a minimum of two to three weeks. You will need this much practice to develop the technique of being able to relax yourself. Each time, do the entire exercise. Be sure you tense and relax each area twice. This will take about one-half hour at first, but after a while you will probably be able to do the exercise in fifteen to twenty minutes. If you can record the instructions, you can do the exercise without having to be interrupted by your own reading.

Exercise 5.2 has two goals. The first is to help you continue to develop an awareness of your own body. Being able to know *if* you are tense, *where* you are tense, and *how* tense you are is a necessary first step toward being able to deal with that tension. You will develop this awareness even further in the next section.

The second purpose of Exercise 5.2 is to develop a relaxation technique, which you can use to help yourself relax whenever you want to. By following the instructions consistently, by repeating the exercise daily until you develop the technique well, and by remembering to use the word RELAX each time you let tension go, you will be building what is called a *conditioned relaxation response*. That is, when the relaxation process has become a skill or habit and when the act of relaxation (letting go of tension) has become connected in your own mind with the word RELAX, you may be able to use the technique and that word to relax yourself whenever you feel tense.

BUILDING BODY AWARENESS

Probably the most common advice people give one another is to "take it easy," or, in other words, to relax. The popularity of such advice undoubtedly reflects our awareness that nervous tension is a major contributor to all sorts of problems, including sexual difficulties, nervous stomachs, headaches, and so on. Despite the common wisdom about taking it easy, people continue to suffer. This is because it is one thing to know you ought to relax and quite another thing actually to do it. For men especially it takes more than someone else's advice to be able to relax. To be able to apply the relaxation technique to your own advantage, to help you relax, you need to develop a more sensitive awareness of your own body; in short, to learn to know when you need it.

The idea of paying attention to your body, and specifically to tension, runs counter to the way men are raised. *Not* paying attention to tension becomes a habit in men. It isn't possible to unlearn this habit very quickly, just as it isn't easy to unlearn any habit. What is involved is a process of learning to substitute one habit for another. In this case, the habit you need to develop involves learning to pay attention to your body. With persistence and practice, you can make gains in this direction.

Exercise 5.3: Developing Body Awareness

It is probably easy for you to see how the kind of extreme tension used in Exercise 5.2 could interfere with any activity, including sexual behavior. What you might not realize, however, is that it does not necessarily take that much tension to cause problems, including sexual ones. Learning to detect lesser levels of tension is more difficult than learning to detect extreme levels. It is a sensitivity that must be developed. It is possible for men to become very sensitive—to learn to detect and deal with even low level tension, which can interfere not only with sex, but with other activities as well, and which, if ignored, can lead to sexual difficulties, high blood pressure, ulcers, and other problems. However, since men learn not to pay attention to such things in their daily lives, learning to detect low levels of tension requires a conscious effort. You will need to make time, in other words, for paying attention to your body, since this no longer comes naturally to you.

> *It might help if you kept a record for awhile as a way of reminding yourself to pay attention to your body now and then. Use the Tension-Relaxation Checklist that follows to do this. Keep it with you when you go places, including to work. If necessary, make a copy and keep it in your wallet or pocket, where you can get to it quickly. In the left-hand column write the date; there are spaces for seven days. Across the top are numbers 1 through 4, and under each number are the headings Time and Tension Spots. Make an effort to pay attention to your own body at least four times a day over the next week. Call each of these times, when you pause to pay attention to your body, a* body check. *This will require only a couple of minutes each time you do it; therefore, it should not interfere with other responsibilities you might have, no matter how busy you are. In fact, if you think you are too busy to take out two minutes four times a day, chances are you are chronically tense and need to develop the relaxation technique for the sake of your own health.*

TENSION-RELAXATION CHECKLIST

For each body check note the time plus all tension spots you discover. Do four body checks each day for seven days.

Date	TIME	1 TENSION SPOTS	TIME	2 TENSION SPOTS	TIME	3 TENSION SPOTS	TIME	4 TENSION SPOTS

Paying attention to your body means just that. Stop what you are doing for a moment and focus on the different parts of your body. Be sure to include each of the following areas in a body check: face, jaw, and neck; shoulders, arms, and hands; chest (breathing) and stomach; buttocks, pelvis, and legs. Notice especially your breathing; is it relaxed and easy, or tight and constricted?

You don't need to find a comfortable or private place to do your body checks. Actually, it is much better if you just pause, wherever you happen to be, and do a body check right there and then. Make sure, however, that it is not always at the same time or in the same place. Be sure to spend a moment focusing on each of the body places before moving on to the next. That way, you build a routine and will not miss anything.

After you finish checking your body, make a note of the time on the Checklist and write a brief description of any tension spots you noticed—places on your body where the muscles seem tense. The following sample should give you an idea.

Date	TIME	TENSION SPOTS
Jan. 1	10 a.m.	Stomach, Jaw, Breathing

The purpose of this exercise is to help you make body awareness (that is, the act of paying attention to your body) part of your everyday life. By the time you have done it every day for one week, you will have made a start in this direction. By going through your Checklist now, you may notice certain patterns, places where tension seems to show up repeatedly. This is important information. If it is your stomach that seems to get tight and tense a lot, you may be on your way to an ulcer if you don't learn to deal with it. If it's your jaw, you may be paving the way for chronic headaches or arthritis, and so forth. As you can see, it is very much in your interest to get in touch with your body.

USING THE RELAXATION TECHNIQUE

Once you have learned the relaxation technique and have developed some sensitivity regarding your own body, what remains is to be able to combine or integrate these two skills in a way that will be helpful to you. This process of integration is actually quite simple. You apply the relaxation technique to reduce tension whenever and wherever you perceive it. This process starts when you realize that one or more parts of your body are tense; in other words, when you notice one or more tension spots. Then, for a brief moment, *increase* (exaggerate) the tension, not as much as in Exercise 5.2, but just a little. Then *think* the word RELAX and let the tension go. It's that simple. Yet, you can probably see now how the skills learned in Exercises 5.2 and 5.3 are so important. These skills are the tools that you need to be able to help yourself. You need to know when you are tense, and where your tension is, and you need to have the conditioned relaxation response at your disposal in order to deal with it.

Exercise 5.4: Applying the Relaxation Technique

For practice in using the relaxation technique to deal with body tension, another chart has been devised for you. The Relaxation Response Record is very easy to use and is really just a convenient way to keep track of the times you do use the relaxation technique and for which tension spots. Using the record will help you to develop the habit of detecting tension and applying the relaxation technique to deal with it.

> *Continue doing body checks several times a day. Each time you detect one or more tension spots, use the relaxation technique to deal with them. Momentarily tense the spot just a bit more; think the word RELAX; and let the tension go. Afterward, make a brief note of it in the Record. There are spaces for twenty-four such notations, but you may want to make up additional sheets*

to be sure that you develop the technique well. Remember, when you do your body check, try to pay attention to many areas of your body, not just one or two. Even if you do discover a tension spot, look for others. Remember also to pay some attention to your chest, to notice any tension you may have there, and the way in which you are breathing.

RELAXATION RESPONSE RECORD

Each time you detect a tension spot during a body check, apply the relaxation technique to it and make a note in the Record.

Date/Time	TENSION SPOT(S)	Date/Time	TENSION SPOT(S)

After you have completely filled out your Relaxation Response Record(s), go through the entries. Look to see if there seems to be any pattern; any places in your body where you detect tension repeatedly. If you can use the relaxation technique consistently, you may be able, in the long run, to reduce the level of chronic tension in one or more parts of you.

SUMMARY

A major complaint expressed by men concerns difficulty in relaxing during their sexual encounters. This chapter approaches the problem of anxiety, in detail, for the first time. The key to dealing with this anxiety involves two separate issues, the first having to do with the attitudes that men are taught to take toward sex. By having all the responsibility for it, men approach sex as a performance, which in turn sets the stage for them to be self-conscious and concerned about how well they are doing. The solution lies in changing both men's and women's attitudes towards sex. By making the quality of the sexual relationship a shared responsibility, the performance anxiety that men experience will diminish.

The second issue that contributes to men's difficulties in dealing effectively with anxiety has to do with yet another attitude they are taught—to suppress such feelings in the interest of being able to be competitive, aggressive, and brave. Anxiety or worry is not something that exists in a person's mind alone; it is also reflected in the state of his or her body. If a man is feeling relaxed, his body will show it, and if he is feeling tense, his body will reflect that tension. To learn to deal with anxiety, men need to develop a new habit of paying attention to, rather than ignoring, their bodies. In this way, they can get in touch with feelings of anxiety when they occur.

Once a man has built a greater degree of body awareness, he is then in a position to apply a specific relaxation technique to help relieve his tension when it occurs. Without this body awareness—of knowing when and where you are tense—the relaxation technique is less useful. The exercises in this chapter are designed largely to accomplish these two tasks (learning the relaxation technique, building body awareness) and integrating them so that you can begin to overcome nervous tension daily. Extending this learning to your sexual relationship is covered in chapter 6.

6 overcoming sexual tension

Dealing with nervous tension in day-to-day living was introduced in chapter 5, leaving the problem of nervous tension in sexual situations until this chapter. There are two reasons for this. First, it seems more difficult to learn to detect nervous tension during a sexual encounter than it is in most other situations. This is because the male sexual script makes it easy for a man to get caught up in the act of performing. At the same time, he will tend to pay less attention to his own feelings, except perhaps those in his genitals. By learning first to detect nervous tension in nonsexual situations, learning to do so in sexual situations may be made easier. One purpose of this chapter is to provide the second step—to help you extend the skill of body awareness to sexual situations.

A second problem in dealing with tension in sexual situations is that it is possible to confuse nervous tension (anxiety) and excitement (arousal). When a person begins to get sexually excited, and especially as he or she nears the point of orgasm, the muscles in many parts of the body, including legs, arms, and back, can become extremely tense. This is not nervous tension. To the contrary, this *buildup* of physical tension is a normal part of the sexual response; it makes the *release* of tension, which is the essence of an orgasm, that much more intense.

Because the buildup and release of physical tension is an essential part of the sexual response of men and women, it does not make sense to try and do away with muscle tension during sex. That would take away from the excitement of the sexual encounter, and it might well prevent orgasm. What does need to be dealt with, however, is nervous tension, or anxiety, in sexual situations.

People who complain about difficulties in relaxing during sex are not talking about the buildup in muscle tension that goes along with getting sexually excited. What they more typically are referring to is a general feeling of uneasiness that they experience from the very *start* of the sexual encounter, which prevents them from enjoying themselves as much as they could. This same sense of uneasiness often causes them, in the long run, to avoid sex altogether, rather than attempt it and be frustrated.

It makes sense that sexual encounters will be more fulfilling when they are approached, or started, with a relaxed, comfortable attitude rather than with a tense, nervous one. When this happens, we are free to experience the buildup of sexual tension and the release of orgasm that follows. A useful goal to pursue, then, would be to be able to *begin* a sexual encounter free of worry, distractions, and other sources of nervous tension. This will, in fact, be our goal here.

SETTING THE STAGE FOR RELAXATION

The first step in the process of overcoming sexual tension is learning to create a situation that is conducive to relaxation. In other words, you need to be able to set the stage in such a way that you will feel at ease, not pent up, at the outset of a sexual encounter. Many people who complain that they are unable to relax and enjoy their sexual relationships seem to overlook the importance of the physical situation in which these sexual encounters take place—things like timing and atmosphere. They also often seem to overlook the importance of the *prelude* to a sexual encounter, the time that immediately precedes lovemaking. These two factors (the physical situation and the prelude) seem to me very important. If one or both are somehow "wrong" for me, my enjoyment of a sexual encounter will be diminished. If the situation is wrong, I will feel uncomfortable or distracted. If I have not had a chance to wind down from a busy day, or if my partner and I have not had an opportunity to relax or play together, I will be pent up or tense. Under such circumstances, I will most certainly not enjoy lovemaking as much as I can (and do) at other times.

When two people are in the process of building a relationship, they often devote a lot of attention to lovemaking. During this initial phase, they not only spend a lot of time making love, but they are also very romantic and playful, and generally take care to set the stage for their sexual encounters. Although some of their encounters may occur suddenly, and without much in the way of a prelude, this tends to happen mainly after they have been apart for a period of time. At such times, sex is a way of getting close—of reuniting—quickly. When they have not been separated, a couple's sexual encounters during the early phases of the relationship tend to follow a romantic prelude. They talk, have fun together, flirt, touch each other in warm and caring ways. Sex then follows this prelude and is very enjoyable for both partners.

As a relationship becomes more established, it also becomes a good deal more complex. Typically, the partners begin to share more than just a sexual relationship, and their responsibilities to each other go beyond sexual pleasure. For example, they may share a home, children, and a family that extends beyond them. Our society looks more or less kindly on the heightened sexual and romantic involvement of couples who are in the building stages of their relationships. Unfortunately, after this initial phase, couples are strongly encouraged to devote themselves to other responsibilities, such as making money, raising children, or tending to family matters. Sexual pleasure, meanwhile, gets a lower priority. Couples are, of course, expected to have a sexual relationship, as well as enjoy certain other pleasures, both alone and together. However, it seems that they are also expected to fit such things into their relationship in between other responsibilities. Their right to have fun, including sexual fun, is given a back seat to their responsibilities. People who challenge these values and put their own pleasure higher up on the list of priorities are often looked on as selfish, misguided, immature, or irresponsible.

But you don't have to neglect, much less give up, a home, children, family, and so on in order to have a fulfilling relationship, sexually or otherwise. You do need to give pleasure something of a priority, however, if you expect to get much of it. So long as fun remains something that must be squeezed into your life, if and when there is time, you will find yourself having very little of it.

Following is a situation in which a good number of couples find themselves during the middle years of their relationship.

> Sex takes place once or twice, sometimes three times a week. It happens late at night, when both partners are feeling tired. They have spent little time together beforehand, for example, talking or doing something they both enjoy. Most likely they have just collapsed in front of the television after the kids are in bed and the last of the chores is finally finished. If they do talk, the topics of conversation may be various problems, or perhaps a decision that needs to be made. The decision to make love, meanwhile, is based largely on whether both partners have enough energy, as well as the inclination, when they finally go to bed. Too often, it is only one of them who really wants it, with the other accepting perhaps a bit reluctantly.

Does the above scene turn you on sexually? Probably not. Does it disturb you? It should. Many people who feel committed to their relationships unfortunately end up in situations very much like this one. The reason is not that they don't care about each other or that they have sexual hang-ups; rather, it is that they have, often without thinking, allowed themselves to put a low priority on their sexual relationship. By giving other matters higher priorities, meaning more time, sex and other forms of fun slowly begin to fall by the wayside.

An outstanding feature of the above scene is that it is not, in a word, sexy. It does not turn you on, and one reason is that it does not include anything like a romantic prelude. There is nothing in it that would lead you to expect that the couple who follows such a pattern would feel close to one another by the time they turn off the television and retire to the bedroom. It is unlikely that their relationship was always this way and unlikely that they took up this sort of pattern suddenly at some point. Instead, the pattern seems to emerge gradually, over a period of years, often without either partner being aware of what is happening. As various other responsibilities gradually consume more and more hours of the day, fun and sex either slip away or else have to fit in under circumstances that are not conducive to enjoyment.

The following exercises ask you to pay some attention to the time you and your partner typically spend together *before* a sexual encounter and how you might rearrange this time to create a more relaxing and enjoyable prelude to sex.

Exercise 6.1: Taking Care of Business

You would probably agree that the middle of a sexual encounter is not the best time to be thinking about the aggravation you had that day at work, the argument you and your partner had yesterday, the children's problems in school, shopping you need to do tomorrow, and so forth. Yet many people find themselves doing just that. Obviously this takes away from whatever pleasure they may derive from lovemaking. It is also one of the main reasons that many people are unable to *start* a sexual encounter in a relaxed, comfortable manner. They are, in effect, too caught up in different sorts of "unfinished business" to be able to relax. This also distracts them from one another and makes it more difficult for them to feel close.

Clearly, trying to take care of business at the same time you make love is a good way to undermine a sexual experience; doing it regularly is a good way to sabotage a sexual relationship. If you want to approach sex with a relaxed rather than a tense attitude, one thing you must be willing to work on is any tendency you might have to carry unfinished business into the bedroom. The following are offered as guidelines in helping you to overcome such difficulties.

> *Don't try to solve all your problems by yourself. When you and your partner are alone together in the evening, don't turn on the television, at least not right away. Instead, set aside half an hour or an hour each night for the two of you to sit and talk about all the "business" facing you. Make an effort to talk about things that are bothering you—finances, work, children, each other, whatever. If something doesn't get settled (which is very likely), put it on the agenda for the following evening. Above all, try to learn to share responsibility for solving problems and to be sources of support for each other when one of you is feeling down in the dumps.*

> *Rather than assuming that everything is fine with your partner, ask her (or him) how she (he) is feeling and if there is anything she (he) is especially concerned about. Doing this can help to establish a pattern of communication and break any tendency to mull over problems in silence.*

> *If you go to bed and find yourself distracted by other business, take a chance and say so. Stop your encounter for a while and talk about whatever it is that is on your mind. Then, if you feel more relaxed, pick it up again.*

> *If the business that gets in the way of your ability to relax in bed has to do with your partner, there is little chance that lovemaking will be fulfilling for you so long as the issue bothering you remains unsettled. Try to talk about it, even if it leads to an argument. Sometimes sex can be much better after the air is cleared.*

Your reaction to the above may be that it is nothing more than common sense (and old-fashioned) advice. It is exactly that. Although there is nothing original in these ideas, they represent sound advice to anyone who desires a better sex life. As simple and "common sense" as they are, few of us are able to follow such guidelines in our day-to-day lives. The more you and your partner are able to do so, the more likely that you will be able to approach sex with a positive attitude.

You and your partner will probably need to work at taking care of business if you want to get the desired results. This will be even more true if your typical pattern leans more toward avoiding conflict or the sharing of concerns. When couples have fallen into such a pattern, the idea of breaking the ice and talking about problems, facing up to issues between them, or sharing responsibilities can be a very frightening proposition. One or both partners may fear that open conflict will lead to a breakup of the relationship. Or each may react to the other's complaint as though he or she were being blamed. Then again, each may feel responsible for finding solutions to the problems and may feel unnecessarily burdened by this responsibility. For all of these reasons, it is important that both you and your partner read this material and make a joint decision whether to try Exercise 6.1. If you both feel that it would be beneficial to your relationship to work on taking care of business, the chances of this exercise being helpful will be considerably greater than if only one of you really wants to do it.

If you, as a couple, decide to go ahead with this exercise, begin by setting aside some time each day when you can start to discuss concerns, complaints, or other problems, and to share responsibility for making decisions. Try to keep the above caution in mind; for instance, it may not be any one person's fault that certain problems exist. The goal of taking care of business is to be able to *share* concerns, as well as the responsibility for their solutions, to settle issues between you, and to give each other emotional support.

You need to give this exercise a good try and to stick with it for a while, especially if you are not used to communicating about problems. For most couples, persistence will lead to positive results. However, after working for a time on making this exercise a regular part of their lives, some couples may find that it does not seem to work. Instead of helping to settle conflicts, talking may lead to more arguments; instead of relaxing them, talking makes them more up-tight. In short, they may discover that communicating, rather than bringing them closer, drives them apart. This can be a sign of a troubled relationship. Such troubles often require the assistance of a trained marital counselor if the people involved are unable to overcome their conflicts and experience a greater degree of intimacy. In the meantime, they may have no choice but to put up with a less than satisfying sex life.

Exercise 6.2: Preludes to Sex

At the beginning of this chapter, we mentioned the important role that the time preceding a sexual encounter plays in the quality of that encounter. The ways in which you and your partner spend this time will influence your sexual interest and the atmosphere under which your lovemaking begins. If you spend time together playing, relaxing, touching, or talking—in other words, if there is a prelude to sex—the chances are that you will look forward to making love and that you will begin to do so feeling relaxed and comfortable with one another. In contrast, if you devote little or no time to getting close, your sexual relationship will probably suffer for it.

Couples often discover the beneficial effects of a romantic prelude when they are in other than a home situation, for example, when they take a vacation together. One reason that sex is often better on such occasions is that the time they spend together before going to bed contrasts sharply with their usual pattern. They have more time to talk, to play, to be romantic, and to get close. As a result, they are more relaxed and look forward to making love.

You can work toward improving the attitude with which you

approach sex by devoting some attention to creating a prelude to your sexual encounters. Experiment with the following guidelines to see how a romantic prelude can affect your sexual relationship.

> *Don't restrict affection to the bedroom. When you feel affection for your partner, express it, using words or gestures, be it in the living room, kitchen, playroom, or backyard, and whether you are alone, with your children, family, or guests. In short, demonstrate your affection to your partner at the time you feel it.*
>
> *Don't limit affection to sex. When sex becomes the only way two people (or one) have of showing affection, one or both often end up resenting it. Sex may be the most powerful way of showing affection and getting close, but it should not be the only way.*
>
> *Work on re-establishing a romantic atmosphere in your relationship. Also, learn to play together. This may feel awkward at first, and you may think it childish or silly. This is because you have let romance and play take a back seat to responsibility in your relationship. Romance is fun, and you may by now have let fun become a low priority. If you work on re-establishing romance, you will be working on putting some of the fun back into your relationship. The exercises in the final section of this chapter may be helpful in this regard.*

Trying to re-establish an atmosphere of romance and playfulness will contribute to your general comfort and ability to relax with your partner. This will, in turn, have beneficial effects on your sexual relationship. In addition to making such general changes, you should work specifically on creating preludes that will be conducive to beginning your sexual encounters in a relaxed manner. The times to do this are those occasions when you (or your partner) feel like having sex. Instead of waiting until you are in bed to start getting close, begin before then. Cuddle up to each other, hold hands, or put your arms around each other. Say some nice things to each other. Try to say and do things to make each other feel good, relaxed, and close. Do things together that you both enjoy. If you are not able to do this or have a great deal of difficulty with it, it should come as no surprise that you are having trouble relaxing and enjoying sex as much as you would like to. It would also be a clear indication that you need to work hard on breaking the ice and rebuilding some sense of intimacy and warmth in your relationship.

As is true for most of the work described in this book, a cooperative effort between two people is more likely to lead to beneficial (and faster) results than is one person working alone. To exist in a relationship, the qualities of intimacy and warmth especially depend upon both partners.

PLANNING FOR RELAXATION

So far, the exercises in this chapter have aimed at helping to clear the way for enjoyable sexual encounters. Taking care of concerns and worries that are sources of distraction during sex and creating a romantic atmosphere before making love will pave the way for you to *begin* a sexual encounter feeling relaxed and close to your partner. Another tool that you can use toward this end is the relaxation technique learned in chapter 5.

By following the relaxation procedure daily, in the long run you can significantly reduce chronic tension, which interferes with your ability to enjoy anything, including sex. A good time to do this is after the chores for the day are done, and after you and your partner have had a chance to sit together and take care of any business that needs to be settled or just talked about. At that point, you can go into your bedroom, or some other quiet place, and take twenty minutes or so to relax your body. It will be time well spent. Use the relaxation technique to do this. If you have recorded the instructions, play the tape and use the tensing-relaxing procedure on each part of your body. If you are particularly tense in some places, repeat the procedure a couple of times in those places after you have gone through the whole exercise.

Finish your relaxation session by lying still for five minutes. Clear your mind of other thoughts and focus attention on your chest and breathing. Let your breathing be easy, relaxed, and deep. Pay attention to the sounds of your own breathing and to the feelings in your chest. Breathe by letting your stomach move in and out. Remember, if you find your mind drifting to other thoughts, bring your attention back to your breathing. This form of meditation has been found to be effective in helping people to overcome chronic tension and to feel refreshed. You may not, however, notice much improvement at first. But if you stick to the procedure, making time for a relaxation session once a day, you should begin to notice a change within a few weeks. You will feel refreshed, less pent up, and ready to spend some time with your partner.

SENSUAL MASSAGE

Besides using the relaxation technique to reduce tension in general, it is possible to apply it during a sexual encounter to increase your sense of comfort. By using it in the context of a *sensual massage,* you may be able to begin your sexual encounters in a manner that is both pleasing and very comfortable.

The purpose of a sensual massage, described in the following exercise, is to allow a couple the opportunity for physically intimate contact, to explore one another on a physical level in new ways, and to help each other to relax and feel good. Although it may lead to more intense sexual contact, it does not have to and can be enjoyed for itself. Couples who include activities like sensual massage in their sexual repertoire report that it results in their feeling closer to one another and it seems to help their ability to enjoy one another in general.

Exercise 6.3: Practicing Sensual Massage

Before beginning this exercise, you and your partner should both read through these instructions completely, or one of you should read and explain them in detail to the other.

Begin by arranging to have an hour or more of uninterrupted privacy. You can do this exercise in your bedroom if you like, but you can also use any other comfortable place, so long as you are sure of privacy. In fact, it may be fun to do it in a place other than your bedroom. Let one of you make it his or her personal responsibility to arrange for a comfortable, romantic atmosphere. If you decide to do the exercise more than once, however, take turns or share this responsibility. Clean up the room and fetch some pillows and blankets, some massage or baby oil, baby powder, and towels. If it is cold, turn up the heat a little for a while. Light a candle or two, put on some soft music, pour a little wine, whatever pleases you and your partner. Your goal in setting up the room is to create a warm, comfortable, and romantic atmosphere. Once you have done this, remove your clothes. Better yet, take turns removing each other's clothes. Be as affectionate as you like, but do *not* try to get each other sexually aroused to any great degree and do *not* start to make love.

Making sure that the surface will be comfortable, let the *man* lie down *on his stomach*. Starting at his head and working slowly downward, let the woman give the man a sensual massage, as described below.

> *When giving someone a sensual massage, one key is to take your time about it. Don't hurry or keep looking at the clock. It is a good idea to do the massage only when you have plenty of time and are not feeling especially tired. When you touch, vary the pressure from very light to hard, but try to use mostly a medium-soft touch. Your goal is not to work out muscle cramps so much as it is to take turns giving and getting pleasure in a relaxed, easy way. You may want to use some massage or baby oil or*

baby powder to make the touching smoother and to make the other person's skin feel good.

Start with the hair and scalp. Run your fingers through the hair several times, slowly, then use your fingertips to lightly massage the scalp. Take your time. Work your way very slowly from the scalp down to the neck. Do the back of the neck and the sides. Take some extra time here because the neck is often a tense spot on a person's body. Then do the shoulders. Don't try to press down too hard for too long, or your hands will get tired. Vary the pressure you use, but use heavier pressure only for brief periods of time.

First do both shoulders at once, using one hand on each, and then do each shoulder using both hands. If you find your fingers or hands beginning to get sore, you are using too much pressure for too long; ease up. As you are massaging your partner, focus your attention on the texture and color of the skin, the contours of the body, the feel of bone and muscle. Pay attention also to the way your partner is breathing. Remember that when a person is relaxed, breathing is easy, deep, and unconstricted. If your partner seems tense, point this out. Do not, however, get into a discussion (or an argument!) about the tension; continue instead with what you are doing.

When you feel you are finished massaging the shoulders, move on to the arms, starting with the upper arms, working your way slowly down to the elbows, the forearms, and the wrists. Do one arm at a time. Use long, light strokes, then firmer strokes. Take one of your partner's hands into yours and gently rotate it to loosen up and relax the wrist. Then do the other one.

Now massage your partner's back. Start high, around the shoulder blades, and work your way gradually down to the waist. Touch it very lightly, then more firmly, then lightly again. If your partner feels tension or pain in one or two specific areas, concentrate on them for a little while. Experiment with different kinds of strokes; short versus long, up-and-down versus side-to-side, straight versus circular. See how your partner responds to these different touches. As you massage your partner's body, notice the way he responds to your touch. This will be most apparent in the way your partner is breathing. If breathing is deep and easy, with an occasional relaxed sigh, he is relaxed.

Pay attention also to the way your partner's body feels. Notice where the skin is smooth and where it is rough, where the body is warm and where it is cool. Feel how the muscles in some places are softer (more relaxed), while in other places they are harder (more tense). Give some attention to the tense places as you discover them, but don't expect that you will be able to remove all the tension from your partner's body.

Now move your hands across your partner's buttocks, lightly at first, then more firmly. Do **not** *touch your partner's genitals, but focus instead on the cheeks of the buttocks. Squeeze them a little and then stroke them lightly again. Gradually work your way down to the thighs. Massage the outsides of the thighs first for a while, then move your partner's legs apart enough for you to be able to massage the insides of the thighs. Try massaging both thighs at once (one hand on each) and then try massaging one thigh with both hands. Use long up-and-down strokes, and then shorter, circular strokes. Experiment with using different degrees of pressure. Find out what pleases and relaxes your partner most, but do not aim at getting him very sexually excited.*

When you feel ready to move on, do your partner's lower legs. These, like the neck, hands, and feet, are often particularly tense at the end of a day, and some brief heavier massaging here might help your partner to relax. Take a somewhat (but not overly) firm grasp of the calf and squeeze the muscles with both your hands to loosen them up. Then stroke the legs lightly, lengthwise, to relax them. After you have finished, ask your partner to roll over onto his back. Now you can massage the feet. As with the hands, take your time and give the feet some extra attention. Do one at a time, massaging the tops, sides, and bottoms. Notice whether the muscles feel loose or tense. Do each toe and the spaces between the toes. Take each foot in both your hands and rotate it to loosen and relax the ankle. Squeeze the foot with both hands, again to loosen up tight muscles. When you finish doing each foot and ankle separately, try massaging both at the same time, using one hand on each. Do this using very light strokes. Use medium-firm pressure, and press your fingertips into the ankles, insteps, and toes.

Moving upward slowly, massage the tops of your partner's legs and thighs. Start with long stroking movements and light pressure, and then focus on smaller areas using a heavier pressure and shorter strokes. Squeeze tense spots to loosen them up and then stroke them lightly to relax them. Take all the time you like. Remember to pay some attention to your partner's reactions—breathing, sighs, and so on. Pay attention also to the body you are touching—its textures and contours.

Now spend a minute touching your partner's genitals. Use a light touch and gentle stroking motions. If this seems to get your partner sexually aroused, fine, but don't make it your goal to get him (her) turned on. This is a sensual massage; it is not really intended to lead to high levels of sexual excitement. Also, do **not** stop the massage here. Concentrate on the way that your partner's genitals feel to you, as well as the reaction that your touching elicits. After you have done this for about a minute, leave this area and move up to the waist and stomach.

Spend some time lightly stroking your partner's stomach and waist. Experiment with different kinds of strokes and with different pressure. Slowly work your way up to the chest. Stroke the breasts, very lightly at first and then a bit more firmly, using small, circular strokes. Use the very tips of your fingers to stroke the nipples and feel their textures. Notice your partner's reactions. Do one breast and nipple at a time, and then try stroking both at once.

Now massage your partner's hands. The hands are places on the body in which tension seems to build up, and having them massaged can be extremely pleasant and relaxing. Do one hand at a time, and take your time. Look at the hand as you stroke it lightly. Hold it in both your hands and massage it a bit more firmly. Do the front and the back. Do each one of the fingers separately, bending and pulling on them to release any tension. Spend some extra time massaging the muscles between the *thumb and forefinger. Experiment with light strokes in between your partner's fingers and see how he reacts.*

The last thing to be massaged is your partner's face. Start with the forehead and work your way slowly around. Don't be in a hurry to finish. Do the temples (some extra time there might be appreciated), the ears, the cheeks, and the chin. When you feel ready, let your partner know that you are finished by giving him a light kiss on the lips.

While the man (in this case) is being massaged, he should try to keep his attention focused on his partner's touch. Every so often, he should shift his attention briefly to his breathing, noting whether it is free and easy or tight and constricted. If it is tight, he should focus on it for a moment, purposefully trying to take deep, easier breaths. As his breathing becomes more relaxed, he can shift his attention back to where his partner is touching him.

As his partner moves on to each new part of his body, the man should note whether the muscles there feel tense or relaxed. If they feel tense, he should ask his partner to pause while he uses the relaxation technique: tense the muscles more, just a little; think the word RELAX; let the tension go.

After the woman has completed her sensual massage, it is her turn to lie down on her stomach while the man uses the same procedure on her, beginning with her hair and scalp.

After your sensual massage, you may go on to further lovemaking if you like, but it is also perfectly fine for your session to end after the massage. If you do go on to further lovemaking, you will be starting with a relaxed, comfortable attitude. This will put you in a position of being able to enjoy the increased intensity of lovemaking much more than you could if you started out feeling tense or distracted.

If you find Exercise 6.3 enjoyable and would like to make it part of your sexual relationship on a regular basis, you may want to experiment with variations of the procedure after a while, to avoid turning it into a routine. There are several good books available that describe the art of sensual massage in greater detail; you can find them in a bookstore.

As long as you remember to focus on your partner's touch and to apply the relaxation technique when necessary, you will in time find yourself becoming more and more relaxed as you repeat the sensual massage. At the same time, you may discover that you don't always want to go on to further lovemaking, but that when you do, your sexual encounters are more fulfilling for both of you than they have been in the past.

PATTERNS OF INTIMACY AND SEXUAL FULFILLMENT

If you have had difficulty in being able to relax and enjoy sex, these exercises and those in chapter 5 can help you. What these programs can *not* do, however, is make you into a sexual machine that will always be up for a sexual encounter. On the contrary, these programs will, if anything, make you more aware of your sexual sensitivities. A critical step along the way to sexual fulfillment is learning more about these sensitivities. Knowing when you are and are not in the mood for sex, and, if you are, what sort of sexual contact you would like, will allow you to get the most from your sexual relationship.

Sex, of course, is one way most couples have of achieving a sense of intimacy in their relationship. Sex is not, however, the only way in which a couple may achieve a feeling of closeness and connectedness with each other. In fact, problems can develop if sex is relied upon too heavily to achieve these goals. There are endless variations of activities that can lead to a sense of intimacy. None of these ways is necessarily "better" than any other. The "best" form of intimacy is the one that meets your needs, and those of your partner, at a given time. Two people will not always want the same thing at the same time, but whenever you and your partner can share a form of intimacy that fits both your needs at that moment, that experience will be immensely satisfying. It will draw you closer together, and it will strengthen the bond of your relationship.

It would be useful if you could devote some time to evaluating the present patterns of intimacy in your relationship seriously. What forms of intimacy do you engage in? Are there many different ways in which the two of you get close, or just a few ways? Has intimacy become channeled into a habit, a single pattern (for instance, sex) that you rely on exclusively, and repeat endlessly, without variation? Do you or your partner feel that you are missing a sense of intimacy in your relationship?

If you do feel that there is something missing, that your sense of intimacy has become dependent upon a narrow, repetitive pattern, you may want to think seriously about changing that. This will take the cooperation and effort of two people, both of whom must want change and each of whom is willing to take some responsibility for it. This means taking risks: making the first move, communicating, being willing to try something new.

Many of the exercises in this book encourage couples to experiment with activities that involve sexual intimacy of various forms. The sensual massage in Exercise 6.3, for instance, is one that couples typically find very enjoyable. Although it may be a less intense experience, in a sense, than a sexual encounter that is more genitally focused, most couples experience it as very intimate in a different way. Once they have had such an experience, they have at their disposal an additional means of getting close. There may well be times when this particular way of being intimate fits both their needs much better than an orgasm.

The advantages of experimenting with new patterns of intimacy and building a repertoire of activities, that is, a number of *intimacy patterns,* is that it leads to a greater sense of satisfaction for both partners and that it takes the burden off genital sex. Consider, for example, a couple who very much desired a feeling of intimacy one evening, but who didn't want (or couldn't have), for one reason or another, a genitally focused sexual encounter. If this couple had come to rely solely on genital sex as a way of getting close, warm, and connected to one another, they would very likely feel frustrated and perhaps angry with one another. On the other hand, if they had alternatives to genital sex available, they might be able to settle on a pattern that would satisfy their needs.

The greater the number of ways that two people have of getting close, the more choices they have and the higher the likelihood that they will be able to find a satisfying pattern of intimacy at any given time. In the long run, they will obviously be closer and feel more connected than couples who restrict themselves to a narrower range of alternatives.

Although the feeling of intimacy can work magic for a relationship, there is really nothing magical about the way intimacy is created. It is created by *doing things* that have the effect of drawing you closer together. Some things that seem to work in this way are doing things to please one another, doing things together that you both enjoy, and sharing thoughts and feelings that you normally keep to yourself. The purpose of the following two exercises is to help you to think in concrete and specific terms about creating intimacy in your relationship.

Exercise 6.4: Caring and Playing

To begin, you and your partner should privately fill out a Caring Behaviors List, shown on the following pages. This should take about half an hour, but it may take longer since you will need to give some thought to being very specific.

CARING BEHAVIORS LIST (MALE)

In the spaces below, write *specific* descriptions of the sorts of things your partner does or can do to make you feel cared for.

1. _____

2. _____

3. ___
4. ___
5. ___
6. ___
7. ___
8. ___
9. ___
10. ___
11. ___
12. ___
13. ___
14. ___
15. ___
16. ___
17. ___
18. ___
19. ___
20. ___

CARING BEHAVIORS LIST (FEMALE)

In the spaces below, write *specific* descriptions of the sorts of things your partner does or can do to make you feel cared for.

1. _____
2. _____
3. _____
4. _____
5. _____
6. _____
7. _____
8. _____
9. _____
10. _____
11. _____
12. _____
13. _____
14. _____
15. _____
16. _____
17. _____

18. _____

19. _____

20. _____

The purpose of filling out a Caring Behaviors List is quite simple. The goal is to provide your partner with a list of specific things that he or she can (or does) do that make you feel cared for.

When people are asked to name the sorts of things that their partners can do to make them feel cared for, they sometimes have a great deal of difficulty being specific. They are prone to saying general things like "showing me affection" or "helping me out." Such statements communicate the general idea of what a person may want in order to feel cared for, but they are vague. If you make statements of this type, don't be surprised if your partner does not understand what you want. These terms often mean different things to different people. What one person feels is giving help might not feel like help to another. Similarly, what one regards as being affectionate may not seem like affection to someone else. This is not because one person has a better idea of what real affection is than another; it is simply a matter of differences in personal preferences. In order for two people to feel cared for by each other, they would need to do the sorts of specific things that each regards as affectionate. In short, the man would need to do the kinds of things the woman finds affectionate, and the woman would need to do the sorts of things the man finds affectionate. The Caring Behaviors List will help you and your partner understand each other's preferences better, so that you can, if you wish to, give the other person what they want.

Use the Caring Behaviors List to write descriptions of as many things as you can think of that your partner can do to make you feel cared for. The behaviors should be specific, clear enough that your partner should have no doubt as to exactly what he (she) can do to please you. For example, you may feel that affection means things like the following:

Giving me a warm hello and a kiss in the morning.
Calling me at work once in awhile, not with a problem, just to say hello.
Coming over and cuddling up next to me on the couch.

Or you may feel cared for when your partner does such things as:

Offer to make me a drink when I get home from work and want to relax.
Take the kids out for a couple of hours so that I can have some time alone every so often.
Surprise me with a little gift (like a nice shirt or a tie) once in awhile.
Cook me a special dinner on a Saturday night.

Each item on your list of caring behaviors should be as specific as the above examples. It is also helpful if the behaviors are all, or mostly all, simple and realistic things. Don't, for example, list "buy me a Rolls Royce," unless your partner is in a position to show caring on such an extravagant level. The things that make us feel cared for really do tend to be small and easily done (if the other person wants to) and things that can be done again and again.

Add behaviors to your list as they occur to you. When you are finished for now, exchange lists and read each other's carefully. Don't be concerned if one list is longer than the other. However, if anything on the list seems vague, so that you don't feel you know exactly what your partner means, ask for details. This is an important step. Don't be too shy to ask each other to be more specific. You need to know as precisely as possible what sorts of things you can do to make your partner feel cared for, and it is your partner's responsibility to make his (or her) desires clear to you.

When you have completed the Caring Behaviors Lists, put them someplace where you both can refer to them as often as you want. At this point, you have it within your means to increase the level of intimacy in your relationship by doing things that make each other feel cared for. The motivation to do this, of course, must come from you and your partner. You needn't turn this exercise into a contest (to see who can do the most caring things), but you can make an effort to do more for each other than you have in the past. Relationships have ups and downs, and when you are experiencing conflict, chances are that you will not be doing as many caring things for each other as you will when things are going well between the two of you. You can check this out by looking at your lists at such times. If you decide, at some point, that you would like to bury the hatchet and get closer, your lists of caring behaviors can be a guideline to doing so. One or the other of you will probably have to be the one to break the ice and make the first move. It might well be worth the risk.

Doing things that make one another feel cared for creates an atmosphere of intimacy in a relationship. This same sort of feeling tends to be created when two people do things together that they *both* enjoy. Sharing pleasant experiences always makes people feel closer to, as well as more comfortable with, each other. The key to creating intimacy in this way, then, is simple: you must share activities and they must be ones that you both enjoy.

To get down to a concrete level again, it would be helpful if you could create a set of guidelines to use if and when you want to increase the level of intimacy in your relationship. To begin, each of you should fill out one of the Pleasant Activities Lists that appear on the following pages.

PLEASANT ACTIVITIES LIST (MALE)

In the spaces below, write *specific* descriptions of activities that you enjoy doing or that you think you might enjoy if your partner did them with you.

1. _____
2. _____
3. _____
4. _____
5. _____
6. _____
7. _____
8. _____
9. _____
10. _____
11. _____
12. _____
13. _____
14. _____
15. _____
16. _____

17. _____
18. _____
19. _____
20. _____

PLEASANT ACTIVITIES LIST (FEMALE)

In the spaces below, write *specific* descriptions of activities that you enjoy doing or that you think you might enjoy if your partner did them with you.

1. _____
2. _____
3. _____
4. _____
5. _____
6. _____
7. _____
8. _____
9. _____
10. _____

11. _____

12. _____

13. _____

14. _____

15. _____

16. _____

17. _____

18. _____

19. _____

20. _____

Beginning with line 1, list as many different activities you can think of that you know you enjoy doing or think you might enjoy doing if your partner did them with you. As with the Caring Behaviors List, be as specific as possible. For example, don't write something vague, such as "going out on a Saturday night." Be more specific: "going to dinner and a movie on a Saturday night"; "going to a concert"; "having friends over for dinner." Make your statements specific enough so that someone reading them would not have any trouble understanding exactly what it is you like to do. In addition, avoid writing once-in-a-lifetime experiences, such as "taking a trip around the world" or "going on a second honeymoon." The problem with such activities is not that they are unpleasant (quite the contrary), but that they are not things you can do easily or often. Your list should contain things that can be done over and over. List as many activities as you can and add more later on if you think of them.

When you have finished filling out your Pleasant Activities List, exchange them with one another and read through them carefully. Don't be concerned if they are not of equal length. However, if any of the things your partner has written seem vague to you, so that you don't feel you understand exactly what activity he (she) is describing, ask for more details. It is your partner's responsibility to be clear and specific about the sorts of activities he (she) likes or might like to do.

Once you have gone through each other's Pleasant Activities List, put them somewhere where you can both consult them at anytime. With these lists, you now have it in your power to create greater intimacy in your relationship if and when you want to. All you need to do is go through your partner's list and look for an activity or two that you also enjoy. Or you can experiment and try an activity that you think you might enjoy doing together. Naturally, this won't include all of the activities your partner has listed, since two people seldom, if ever, have similar tastes in everything. Moreover, there is nothing at all wrong with doing things that you like without your partner. In fact, the more you each feel free to do both sorts of things—share pleasant activities and do fun things alone—the closer and more fulfilling your relationship should be.

Exercise 6.5: Sharing and Intimacy

Another sort of activity that seems to lead to a feeling of intimacy within a relationship has to do with sharing things about yourself that you do not normally share with others. When you are able to be open with your thoughts and feelings in this way, it does two things: it makes the other person feel special and it makes the other person special to you. You become, in a word, attached to that person who listens sympathetically and with interest to your disclosures of personal information. If your own openness is returned, so that your partner shares with you as well as you with him or her, your mutual attachment becomes a bond between you. This is a different sense of intimacy than the one that results from doing pleasant things together, and it is different, too, from the feeling that comes from having sex.

To work toward creating a sense of intimacy through openness and sharing, set aside some time (at least one hour) when you and your partner can be alone in a relaxed atmosphere where you can talk. To mark this as a special time between you, it might be a good idea to go out. If you have children, arrange for a sitter for an hour or so; it will be worth the investment. You needn't go anywhere expensive. Rather, go someplace comfortable where you can relax together for a while and have a conversation without being overheard.

It may seem awkward at first, and you both may be uncomfortable about setting up these special circumstances. You may also be understandably nervous about the prospect of being open and sharing "private" information. You might begin, therefore, by talking to each other about these very feelings. Take turns telling the other person how you felt about going out like this and how you feel about the idea of sharing thoughts and feelings that you normally keep to yourself. Try to be honest. If you feel uncomfortable and nervous, take a chance and say so. Finally, share your concerns about being open with each other. Most people have such concerns. For example, what sorts of reactions would you not *like to get from being open? How would you like your partner to react to your openness? What sorts of thoughts and feelings are you most hesitant to share?*

The person listening should do just that: listen attentively and quietly. This is not the time to make the person talking feel uncomfortable or defensive by asking a lot of questions, or guilty by being asked why he or she hasn't been open about this before. Third degrees and accusations like this are likely to get you nowhere fast. They create bad feelings and drive people apart. Being an unsympathetic listener is the best way to discourage someone else from being open to you.

After you are able to share your feelings (in this case, your feelings about being open), notice how this makes you feel. Chances are if the other person really is sympathetic and interested, you feel good after talking. You probably feel relaxed, even refreshed, and have warm feelings about your partner. Most likely you appreciate the support that comes from sympathy and interest in you.

This is one example of being open. If this sort of sharing of feelings is nothing unusual for you, well and good. On the other hand, if it feels like a new and different experience, you and your partner probably are not accustomed to being open with each other; you might be interested in learning to do so. To continue developing this pattern of intimacy in your relationship, you both will need to take some modest risks, to push yourselves to share thoughts and feelings you have been afraid to share for one reason or another.

If both of you are able to take risks, you can in time build a stronger bond between you. Begin by talking about your concerns. Specifically, tell each other what might have made you hesitate to share certain things in the past. Some of these reasons might have to do with your own personality; others might concern reactions you were afraid you would get if you were open. Try to identify the general nature of the thoughts and feelings you find hardest to share. Consider the following list.

- Fear
- Nervousness
- Shame
- Loneliness
- Discouragement
- Depression

- Sadness
- Anger
- Resentment
- Jealousy
- Weakness
- Pride

The kinds of feelings you need to share are almost always related to some *event* in your life, either past or present. For instance, something happens that causes you to feel fear.

However, rather than being open about it, you may either choose not to talk about it at all, you may talk about the event but not the feelings, or you may lie about your true reaction. The reactions you keep to yourself or lie about will almost certainly be ones you are ashamed of. Being able to share these feelings with another person—to open up this side of yourself to someone else—is one way to build a sense of intimacy. It is also an important way that you can get support and not feel as though you have to go through life's rough spots all alone.

You and your partner should continue to set aside some special time, say once a week, when you can be alone together and talk about yourselves. Use this time to experiment, at your own pace, with sharing thoughts and feelings that you would normally keep to yourself. See how this, in turn, makes you feel and what effects it has on your sense of connectedness to your partner.

SUMMARY

The purpose of this chapter is to provide a set of guidelines that can be applied to helping you overcome difficulties in being able to relax and enjoy your sexual relationship to the fullest. The specific goal is to help get you into a position of being able to begin your sexual encounters with a positive attitude: feeling relaxed, comfortable, and close to your partner. To accomplish this, several factors are emphasized. Sex is something that needs, in a way, to be prepared for. Conflicts and distractions that are carried into the bedroom, for instance, are likely to have negative effects on the quality of a sexual encounter. Similarly, it is more likely that you can approach sex with a positive attitude if lovemaking follows a romantic prelude and if it takes place in a romantic, relaxed atmosphere.

The pressures of day-to-day life and the increasing responsibilities that couples take on during the long middle years of a relationship often cause them to let fun, including sexual fun, slide lower and lower on their list of priorities. As a result, it takes effort and determination to make changes that are conducive to a better sexual relationship. There is a need to make time to talk and to get close, and this means shifting priorities a bit.

Besides establishing guidelines to help set the stage for relaxation, Exercise 6.3 gives you a way to apply the relaxation technique described in chapter 5 in a sexual situation. By using this technique during a sensual massage, both you and your partner have the opportunity to share a relaxing sexual experience; one that can, if you like, be a prelude to a more genitally focused encounter.

The last section of this chapter concerns the relationship between sexual fulfillment and the overall quality of your relationship. A sexual relationship does not flourish when it is cut off from the rest of the relationship or when it becomes the sole means a couple has of achieving intimacy. Rather, sex is more fulfilling when it is *part* of a relationship that has a certain degree of intimacy to it. Such intimacy is not accidental; it is something created by the way a couple treats one another, by the kinds of things the partners do together, and by the amount of sharing they do. It is in your power to create intimacy, if you both wish, and to create an atmosphere in which your sexual relationship can flourish. What is required is the motivation and a certain willingness to take risks.

7 overcoming fears of women

The simplest and most direct way to tell whether you have a fear of women is to pay attention to your own reactions when you are around women you find sexually attractive, especially if there is a possibility for sexual contact. If you have followed the exercises in chapter 5, you should be able to detect if and when you get tense or anxious in such situations. Such fears can be mild or severe. Many men have mild fears of women of one sort or another. In the more severe forms, men who are fearful of women will avoid them (especially those they find sexually attractive) as much as possible, sometimes completely. When they either can't (or don't want to) avoid women, these men experience *anxiety symptoms*. Such symptoms may include heartburn or nausea, stuttering, profuse sweating, and a fast, pounding heartbeat. Milder forms of discomfort are associated with less severe anxiety symptoms—sweaty palms, "butter-flies" in the stomach, occasional difficulty speaking fluently, and so on. We will call this form of fear of women, whatever its intensity, *sexual shyness*. It has to do with being generally uncomfortable around women to whom you are attracted.

A second form of fear is more specific and may or may not occur along with the kind described above. This appears as a discomfort about looking at or touching women's bodies, especially their genitals. Again, it can vary in intensity from strong feelings of anxiety and disgust, at the one extreme, to mild feelings of uneasiness at the other. We might call this form of fear a *sexual phobia,* since it is somewhat more specific and limited than sexual shyness.

SEXUAL SHYNESS

This type of discomfort around women is often linked to a fear of rejection or, what amounts to the opposite side of the same coin, an excessive concern with the approval of others. Underlying this form of woman phobia is an expectation in the man that his interest in a woman will go unrewarded—she will not be interested in return. He may fear that he will be rejected by the woman because of something he imagines he lacks (or does lack), for instance, money, status, looks, or sophistication. If he has experienced sexual problems, he may fear that his initial interest may be accepted, but that he will be rejected later on by the woman if he has sexual difficulties (that is, when his sexual performance is not what he imagines she would want) when he is in bed with her. Finally, he may fear that she will disapprove of his interest, for one reason or another.

These are all fears of some sort of *external punishment,* that is, a punishment you expect to come *from the woman.* There may also be an expectation of some form of *internal punishment,* which is to say a punishment that comes *from you* rather than the woman. You may expect that you will feel sinful, dirty, or otherwise badly about yourself for expressing a sexual interest. Or you may be critical of yourself if your sexual interest is accepted, but your performance doesn't meet your own demands.

Exercise 7.1: Understanding Your Sexual Shyness

Consider your particular form of shyness for a moment. Imagine the last few times you have been around a woman you were attracted to. Try to recreate one such experience in your own mind and to get in touch with the feeling of anxiety you have in such situations.

Try to think of your sexual shyness as a fear. Specifically, try to think of it as an expectation you have that something negative will result from your sexual interest if you express it or try to act on it.

Try now to identify the specific nature of your expectation by answering the following questions, checking off all answers that seem to apply to you.

1. Is your expectation for internal punishment (bad feelings you would have about yourself), external punishment (rejection by the woman), or both?

    ____ internal only   ____ external only   ____ both

2. What sort(s) of external punishment do you expect?

    ____ (a) A woman will think badly of me for expressing a sexual interest in her.

    ____ (b) A woman won't think badly of me for expressing a sexual interest, but she won't be interested in me.

    ____ (c) My sexual interest might be reciprocated, but the woman might reject me because of my sexual performance during lovemaking.

3. What sort(s) of internal punishment do you expect?

    ____ (d) I will feel ashamed of myself for trying to seduce a woman.

    ____ (e) I won't reject myself for expressing a sexual interest, but I would reject myself if my interest is accepted and I don't perform the way I want to.

If you checked answers (a) and/or (d), your negative expectations probably have to do with feeling guilty about sex. Most likely this reflects an attitude developed early in your life that sex was somehow wrong or sinful, that "good" people didn't do that sort of thing, and that you should be ashamed of sexual thoughts or wanting to have sexual contact with a woman.

If you checked answers (c) and/or (e), your negative expectations reflect *sexual performance anxiety* on your part. You don't believe that it is wrong to have sexual feelings, but you fear that you will not perform the way you want to and as a result will be rejected by the woman, by yourself, or both. This sort of fear contributes substantially to sexual dysfunctions in men, especially to erection problems. Worrying about "failing" only makes the situation more tense, so that sexual difficulties end up being a sort of self-fulfilling prophecy.

Checking answer (b) suggests a lack of self-confidence in a different sense. Men who feel that they have little to offer tend to hold expectations that the women they like will not like them. In some cases this expectation may be realistic (based on actual experience of being continually rejected), but often it has to do with feelings of inferiority that come from childhood and adolescence. Frequently, men who check answer (b) have not actually had the experience of being repeatedly rejected by women; they only believe that they would be if they tried.

From Exercise 7.1 you can see that there are several different reasons why a man might choose to avoid women and that one man's sexual shyness may not be based on the same sorts of fears as another man's. How you go about overcoming your shyness depends to some extent on which type(s) you seem to have. If your problem is one of feeling guilty (and being inhibited) about your own sexuality, the exercises in chapters 2 and 4 may be helpful to you. Avoiding women because of intense feelings of inferiority and unattractiveness is, in general, more effectively dealt with through counseling than a self-help book, and you may want to consider this option. If you are at a point where you do not even attempt to date women you are attracted to for fear that you are not worthy enough or attractive enough, it is unlikely that a self-help book can give you the kind of support you need right now, but you can get help from a personal counselor. In addition, you may need to explore in some depth the causes for your sense of inferiority and devise an individualized treatment program that will help you to develop your social confidence one step at a time.

Sexual performance anxiety (see chapter 5) is frequently the key factor underlying sexual shyness. This is especially true for men who have experienced a sexual dysfunction, for example, problems with erections or quick ejaculations. Men often take such difficulties as personal failures, signs of inadequacy. A fear of "failing" during a sexual encounter leads many men to avoid sexual situations. For some, this means avoiding women, period, or at least avoiding all but the most formal sorts of contact with them. Other men don't give up relationships with women altogether. Instead, they move from having sexual relationships to having platonic (friendship) relationships with women to whom they are sexually attracted. In this way they avoid what they consider to be risky sexual encounters, but they are still able to maintain relationships. This option may be more desirable than the first; it may, for instance, prevent extreme social withdrawal. In the long run, however, it tends not to be very satisfying, since these men are left feeling sexually frustrated, and as time goes on their self-confidence erodes.

Sexual performance anxiety has two possible sources. One is a fear that a woman will reject you if and when you "fail" during a sexual encounter. Failure in this sense, as we said, usually means either not getting (or keeping) an erection, or ejaculating prematurely. A second source of performance anxiety has less to do with the woman; it is an expectation that you will get down on *yourself* for not performing the way you think you should.

Performance anxiety is linked in a very direct way to the male sexual script and the sexual myths discussed in chapter 1.

Sexually and otherwise, men are expected to be rugged, which means that they are not supposed to have sexual difficulties. This standard does not generally apply to women as severely as it does to men because women's sexuality has always been thought to be more sensitive. Although women may be subject to performance anxiety (and probably are more and more), it would still be fair to say that it would be less embarrassing, more acceptable, for a woman to admit that she is not comfortable enough with a man to go to bed with him yet, or that she doesn't usually reach orgasm the first few times she goes to bed with a new partner, than it would be for a man to turn down a sexual invitation, or to have trouble keeping an erection the first few times he went to bed with a woman.

Because of their need to be (or at least to seem) sexually expert, men don't talk much about their sexual difficulties, but they have them for sure. A number of women have recounted experiences they have had with men reaching orgasm too quickly or not being able to maintain an erection, especially during their first few sexual encounters with them. As one woman told this familiar tale, a man who did not get an erection the first time she went to bed with him said to her, "I don't understand it. This has never happened to me before." Tired of hearing this line, the woman replied, "That's funny, it seems to happen to me often."

It is probably fair to say that men expect entirely too much of themselves sexually, especially during the early stages of a relationship. They are usually eager to prove their virility to a new partner, by impressing her with their sexual hardware and skill. This is just another example of the way in which men swallow the old myths about male sexuality, as though being a sexual machine was something to be proud of. Owning up to the fact that you are not a machine but a sensitive human being and that your sexual performance will not always be the same will go a long way toward reducing sexual performance anxiety. It will do so by making it less of a personal catastrophe in your own mind to experience sexual difficulties.

As for fears that a woman will kick you out of bed because you don't get or keep an erection or because you reach orgasm quickly, there is little basis for this. Even if men don't admit it, women know the truth—men do have difficulties, a lot more often than they are willing to admit. I personally have never spoken with a woman who felt she had rejected a man solely because of a sexual dysfunction on his part. On the other hand, I have spoken with men who believed that this was why they were rejected. Although in some rare cases this may have been true, there were probably other reasons for the rejection, which these men preferred to ignore, choosing instead to blame it on their sexual "inadequacy."

The great majority of women seem to have a patient and sympathetic attitude toward male sexual problems and they don't think less of a man who does experience difficulties. Moreover, male sexual dysfunction is rarely the sole reason why a woman might break up a relationship she otherwise finds rewarding. Women's main sexual complaints about men do not, in fact, concern erections or ejaculations at all. Rather, they have to do with the feeling that there is too little affection and intimacy in the relationship as a whole, too little foreplay, and virtually no afterplay as part of the sexual relationship.

Finally, whereas the man who experiences a sexual problem usually blames himself, feeling that he is inadequate or inferior, it is not at all uncommon for his partner to blame herself for it. Feeling that she is not attractive enough, or skilled enough, or perhaps that she is being too demanding are concerns commonly expressed by women whose men are experiencing sexual dysfunctions. The irony in this sort of situation is cruel; a man and a woman both believing the myths about male sexuality and expecting too much, each blames his- or herself. To top it off, often neither one talks to the other about his or her feelings, but they go on suffering in silence, feeling more and more unhappy with themselves and their relationship.

Overcoming sexual shyness based on performance anxiety has a good deal to do with changing your attitudes about male sexuality. Also helpful, however, are new experiences with women. If you are one of those men who has avoided all romantic contact with women for fear of having sexual difficulties, but you still have platonic relationships with a few women, a good *first step* for you to take would be to date again without feeling intensely anxious. It would be a good idea, however, if you could make a firm decision, *beforehand,* that you will *not* go to bed with a woman on these dates even if she makes it clear that she would like to do that. If you think this makes sense, but you feel that it would be difficult for you to set this limit with a woman who expressed a sexual interest in you (that is, to turn her down), the exercises on Sexual Communication in chapter 3 will help you. Except for this limit on the extent of sexual contact, these should be "real dates" with women you are sexually attracted to. Try to get beyond the platonic stage while still not going to bed. Try to let it be known that you are attracted and try to find out if your feelings are reciprocated. Kissing, holding, and so forth are completely acceptable on such occasions, although you may want to exercise some self-restraint if you feel this could end up being very frustrating for the two of you.

If dating brings on severe anxiety symptoms, and/or if you have avoided women altogether, here are two suggestions. First, learn the relaxation technique described in chapter 5 and use it to help relax yourself before and even during a date. Second, move even more slowly than the pace described above for men who have maintained platonic relations and who feel less tense. You still need to move beyond the formal, sexless stage in male-female relations, but in your case a comfortable platonic relationship would be a step forward.

After learning the relaxation technique, try asking a woman that you like, but are not intensely attracted to sexually, to take a lunchtime stroll with you, go window shopping, or have lunch. If you do go somewhere together, choose a place that appeals to you and is comfortable, but that does *not* have a very romantic atmosphere. There is probably no way that you can avoid all anxiety when taking this first step. But as far as breaking the ice is concerned, there is simply no way to do it but to do it. Using the relaxation technique, choosing a woman you like but are not highly turned on by, and selecting a comfortable but nonromantic setting for these early dates should at least reduce your tension.

It may take some time for you to overcome your initial anxiety about being with a woman, even if you are not terribly attracted to her. Do not wait, however, for your tension to disappear completely before moving on to the next step. You should proceed just as soon as you feel that your anxiety has been reduced to manageable proportions. In other words, push yourself a little; it may take too long to wait for your anxiety to disappear completely. This *second step* is for you to repeat the above procedure, only this time with at least one, and preferably several, women to whom you are more sexually attracted *and* who you think might be attracted to you. Approach them in much the same way, suggesting the same sorts of activities (a walk, lunch, or an after-hours drink), and once more, choose places that are comfortable but not particularly romantic. Assuming that you really are sexually interested in these women, your level of tension should jump when you first attempt this step. This is to be expected and is perfectly normal. Use the relaxation technique again to help keep your nervousness within tolerable limits.

Once you have accomplished the above, you will be in just about the same place as those men who began with a less severe sexual shyness than you. You may then proceed to the step described earlier, to begin dating with the understanding (in your own mind) that you will not yet go to bed.

Once you are at the point where you are again able to date women to whom you are attracted (and who are attracted to you) and can engage in some form of physical affection, your sexual shyness should be much less severe, and you are ready for the *third step*. Since your particular fear is rooted in performance anxiety, one way, and perhaps the best way, to deal with it is to confront it more or less directly when it happens. What you expect and fear is that you will be rejected by a woman because you will experience some sexual difficulty. This fear not only makes you shy away from sex, it also makes it more likely that you *will* experience a sexual dysfunction when you have a sexual encounter. Obviously, one way to deal with this expectation is to beat it to the punch, so to speak. You can do this by disclosing the fact that you have experienced sexual difficulties in the past, and that you have, as a result, become nervous about sexual contact. You can do this, moreover, *before* you ever get to the point of having a sexual encounter.

Full disclosure of your sexual anxieties in advance may make sense to you, and you may decide to go ahead and do it. On the other hand, most men seem to shrink from this prospect. They feel it would be too embarrassing or too awkward to talk about their past sexual experiences and current fears with a woman they were attracted to, but had not as yet been intimate with. For these men, an alternative to disclosure is discussed later on.

If you do decide to tell a woman about your fears ahead of time, you should make your disclosure only to a woman you feel sexually attracted to, who you think returns the feeling, and with whom you feel reasonably comfortable. Although it usually takes people sometime to feel comfortable with one another, this can also happen at times on a first date, and it can happen with someone you never expect to see again. When you do decide to talk, you might disclose three things: the fact that you find the woman you are with sexually appealing, the general nature of your past sexual difficulties, and the fear of getting sexually involved, which reflects your fear of "failing." The following exercise may be useful as a guide in accomplishing these goals.

Exercise 7.2: Sexual Self-Disclosure

Let's apply the behavioral rehearsal technique (see chapter 3) again to give you some practice in disclosing your sexual history and relieving some of the anxiety that goes along with that situation. Imagine the following scene, making it as real as possible in your imagination. Make sure you say all of *your* lines *out loud*.

> *You are with a woman you find very sexually attractive. You have had a very pleasant evening together and now the two of you are alone in your apartment. You are sitting next to her on your living room couch. As you talk, imagine yourself moving a bit closer to her. She smiles. As you look at her, you are aware of how very sexually attractive you find her. Look at her now and say to her* **out loud:** *"I think you're very attractive."*
>
> *If saying the above line caused you to feel tense, repeat it, out loud, before proceeding.*
>
> *Imagine that the woman smiles at you again and thanks you for the compliment, then adds that she thinks you're attractive, too. Reply to her,* **out loud:** *"Thank you. I'm really glad to hear that you like me, too. I really am attracted to you, but to tell you the truth I'm feeling sort of nervous right now. If you're up to listening, I think I'd like to tell you about it."*
>
> *Repeat the above lines again, out loud. Imagine as best you can that there is a woman beside you, listening to you. Change the words to suit yourself, but get the same message across. When you feel reasonably comfortable (don't expect to feel completely comfortable), proceed.*
>
> *Imagine now that the woman leans toward you just a bit. She says that she would be glad to listen. Imagine yourself looking at her, and say,* **out loud:** *"Well, the problem is I've had some sexual difficulties in the past, and it's made me sort of scared to get sexually involved."*
>
> *Repeat the above line again, just to see how it feels to say it, and then proceed, saying,* **out loud:** *"The truth of the matter is that I'm afraid I'll have the problem again and that would be very embarrassing."*
>
> *Repeat the last line again, out loud, while imagining as best you can that you are saying this to a woman.*

Well, how was that? Tense? That's okay. After all, you have just told a woman that this is something you *are* nervous about! However, getting the issue out in the open may make things somewhat easier later on.

It is a rare woman who will reject a man who is honest with her, especially when it is about something so vulnerable as his sexuality. However, most women, like most men, are far from comfortable or sophisticated when it comes to the topic of sex. Therefore, although it is doubtful that a woman will feel badly about you or put you down for talking about yourself, what is likely is that she will feel embarrassed. She may feel this way simply because she isn't used to talking about sex and doesn't know what to say. Or she may feel put on the spot, thinking that you want something from her that she might not want to give you. The less time you've known a woman and the less intimate you've been with her, the more likely it is that disclosure will get you these sorts of reactions.

If you choose to disclose your sexual concerns and if this works out well for you, the next step is to go ahead and have a sexual encounter if the opportunity arises. Accept the fact that you may again experience difficulties, at least the first few times you go to bed. Remember that disclosure may relieve anxiety, but it is seldom a cure. Concentrate on being able to get close and have fun together, rather than spending your time lying there worrying about your penis. Resist any urge to stop a sexual encounter if and when you experience your old difficulties. Instead, focus on your lover, on pleasing her, and on being pleased in as many ways as you can. Experiment a little, for instance, with a sensual massage or a vibrator. Later on, if a particular woman is interested in helping you to work on whatever it is that concerns you, the two of you can read the relevant self-help program, described in later chapters.

When I first began to work with single men who were experiencing sexual difficulties, my inclination was to advise them to disclose something about their past experiences and their concerns to a woman they were attracted to, at a point when a sexual relationship seemed a possibility. My thought was that disclosure might help to reduce performance anxiety. For those men who found themselves having relationships in which they felt cared for, this strategy, if tried, often did seem to help. In general, it worked to strengthen, not weaken, the relationship, and they reported that sex, when it later happened, was less stressful and more enjoyable.

But, as I mentioned earlier, to most men the idea of disclosure seems equally, if not more, frightening than the idea of having difficulties during a sexual encounter. Many men I work with say that it would be just too embarrassing to admit to having sexual concerns in advance of any sexual contact. Also, not all men feel comfortable enough about a woman—that is, they don't know her well enough—to risk sharing such intimate and sensitive information about themselves early in a relationship. Then again, many express a fear that a woman might feel embarrassed or put out by being told about a man's sexual problems.

Perhaps there is little truth behind these fears, but the fact that a good many people express them is a convincing argument that disclosure, for some men, may not be the best strategy for reducing anxiety. I am now inclined to encourage men to use their judgment—to decide against or for disclosure on the basis of the *particular* circumstances, which means deciding on the basis of the *particular* woman. My thinking has been reinforced, by reports from men who have tried it, that things can work out just as well if you simply take the risk and go to bed with a woman you are attracted to when an appropriate opportunity arises.

Among those men who choose the take-the-risk strategy, the best results seem to occur for those who have changed their attitudes about themselves, specifically their attitudes about their own sexual functioning. Men who have come to accept their sexual sensitivities and who do not take variations in their sexual performance as signs of personal weakness seem always to do better than those who are still hung up about their masculine image.

John was twenty-six years old and single. He had been sexually active from ages twenty-two to twenty-four, but he had avoided women since then because of his embarrassment over sexual difficulties. When he was dating, he had a few different relationships, and sexually these were very disappointing to him. Most of the time he did not get an erection; other times he would get one, but it would subside before he could complete intercourse. After attending a few sessions of a male sexuality group that I was running, he recognized that performance anxiety was mainly responsible for his difficulties. He recalled that he would feel very tense as soon as a sexual encounter began, and he realized that it was his erection he was worried about. His worrying, in turn, had ruined his chances of getting or keeping an erection.

John learned to use the relaxation technique and followed a procedure much like the one outlined earlier in this section. After a month he was dating again and feeling pretty comfortable about it. At that point, he knew, the possibility of a sexual encounter—his first in two years—lay ahead of him. Understandably, he was nervous about taking this next step. On the other hand, he had recently met a woman he found very attractive, felt comfortable with, and who seemed very interested in him. We discussed the idea of disclosing his past problems and his current fears about sexual involvement to this woman before going to bed with her. Then we tried out some behavioral rehearsal exercises like the one in Exercise 7.2.

The next week John came to the group session and announced that he had a very pleasant sexual encounter with this woman. Contrary to disclosing his fears, as he had planned to do, he chose instead simply to go ahead and have sex. Although he was very excited and got a strong erection, he lost it after a while, but not until he had at least had an opportunity to enjoy a lot of foreplay and a minute or so of intercourse. At the point when his erection subsided, he did not get upset and stop the lovemaking;

he and his partner continued, doing things for each other that did not require an erect penis. He also recalled having thought to himself, "I'm sensitive. I have a right to be impotent."

Clearly, John's attitudes about his own sexuality had changed a lot, and this helped him feel free to take a risk, sexually speaking. After some initial difficulties, his erection problem gradually improved. When I last saw him he was still having occasional problems with losing his erections, but this did not upset him or otherwise interfere with his enjoyment of his sexual relationship.

As well as John's case worked out, it should not be taken to mean that the solution to all sexual dysfunctions is simply to go to bed with somebody. It is true that reassessing your attitudes toward your sexual performance and your expectations toward an end of being more patient and less critical of yourself can help to reduce performance anxiety. Sometimes this is enough to "cure" the problem, but not always. Many dysfunctions really require, in addition to attitude changes, the cooperative efforts of yourself and a willing, caring partner. Later chapters provide some step-by-step programs for doing this.

SEXUAL PHOBIAS

The second type of fear concerning women has to do with a dislike of, or discomfort with, the female body. Rarely does a man feel uncomfortable about the entire female body; usually it is the genitals specifically that arouse feelings of discomfort. In its milder forms, men who suffer from such a "genital phobia" may be aware only of the fact that they do not enjoy touching, or perhaps even looking at, a woman's genitals. In the more severe forms, genital-phobic men may experience intense anxiety symptoms, including strong reactions of disgust and nausea when attempting to look at or touch female genitals.

Sometimes such anxiety reactions are be based in reality, for example, when a partner whose personal hygiene or grooming is poor. In addition, some men report that their discomfort began only after the woman's physical appearance had changed in some way, for instance, by putting on a lot of weight. If your own discomfort seems linked to such an issue, and if it seems that the problem could be solved by your partner doing something about her hygiene or appearance, you ought to discuss your feelings with her before proceeding any further with this program. Personal hygiene and weight are things that a person can change, at least to some degree, and if this would make you more comfortable your partner may be willing to do something to please you. But if your partner changes and you don't become more comfortable, or if it seems that your discomfort does not have to do with things about your partner's body that she could change, then following-through with this program can help you to overcome your fears.

Men who suffer from a genital phobia (a general feeling of discomfort about female genitals, breasts, or both) often seem to have certain things in common, such as an exceptionally strict, demanding, and rigid upbringing. Somewhere in their youth, these men developed a nervous or tense attitude toward sex in general, and toward women in particular. Whereas most adolescents are told that sexual activity before adulthood (or marriage) is wrong, these men often seem to have gotten the added message that it is dirty, disgusting, or sinful. Later, as adults, they often experience shame over masturbation, guilt over sexual fantasies, and a real hesitation to let themselves be sexual (sexy), in addition to their genital phobia. In other words, it seems that a genital phobia rarely appears alone, but is more typically one part of a larger negative attitude toward sex that was learned in the course of growing up.

With regard to discouraging sex, the parents of men who suffer from this phobia appear to have overdone it a bit. Overcoming a genital phobia, therefore, means overcoming deeply ingrained negative attitudes, and this generally takes some time, plus a real desire to change. You may begin to overcome a genital phobia by attempting to change your attitudes toward sex, as well as some of the other difficulties that often go along with this problem. The exercises in chapters 2 and 4 can help you to do this. In addition, the relaxation technique in chapter 5 will be useful, and you should learn it before going on with this program.

The procedure to help you overcome discomfort about the female body is called *desensitization*. Basically, the idea is to teach a fearful person to relax, and then to have him approach whatever it is he fears in a gradual, stepwise manner. For example, if you were afraid of (uncomfortable with) heights, you would be taught how to relax yourself and then, as a first step in "desensitizing" you to this fear, you would be asked to stand on a short footstool. Later on, you might be asked to relax yourself and then walk up half a flight of stairs and look down, and so on. The final goal might be to get you to feel comfortable dining at the top of the tallest building in your city, but it would be accomplished by moving a step at a time while having you relax.

This type of procedure can be used to overcome a discomfort with the female body. First, however, you need to learn how to relax yourself. Once you have learned the relaxation technique, a conscientious effort to follow-through with the next series of exercises can help you to overcome your phobia.

Exercise 7.3: Letting Yourself Look

After using the relaxation technique to reduce any nervousness you may be feeling, go to a bookstore or newsstand and purchase several soft-core pornographic magazines, such as *Playboy,* that have pictures of nude women in them. Make sure that you do this for yourself; don't ask someone to do it for you. Keep the magazines handy, at home and not hidden. In privacy, and starting out with about five minutes a day, look at the pictures of the women. Shift your attention back and forth among the different parts of their bodies, including the genitals. However, avoid any tendency to look exclusively at the genitals.

If looking at female genitals in the magazine photos makes you feel uncomfortable, tense, or disgusted, quickly try to shift your attention to some other part of the body and keep it there until the tension decreases. If this does not reduce your discomfort, close the book, tell yourself to RELAX (as you learned to do in chapter 5), and then try looking some more.

Naturally, if you find that looking at the pictures in the magazines gets you turned on, that's fine. It is possible, however, that this won't happen at first. It is also possible that you will get only a little turned on and that you could mistake such slight feelings of sexual arousal for feelings of nervous tension. Try not to make this mistake—pay attention to your body and decide whether you are feeling anxious or excited.

Remember that during this early phase of the exercise, it is very important that you avoid any tendency to focus your attention exclusively on the women's genitals, but to look at them alternately with other parts of their bodies. Notice their faces, hair, and skin, their arms, legs, hands, and feet. Compare their figures, their thighs, ankles, and so on. Notice that the genitals, like breasts, are a part of the women. Remember also to use the close-the-book-and-relax procedure to ease any tension. Finally, be sure to do some looking every day.

When you feel comfortable with the first step, purchase a second batch of magazines. First, spend some time looking through the pictures in the usual way—not focusing exclusively on any one part of a body, but more or less taking it all in. Again, try to get a sense of the way a woman's breasts and genitals are parts of a whole person, not things that exist alone. When you feel comfortable doing this, shift your attention slightly so that you do begin to focus more on the breasts and genitals. If and when you begin to have any negative reactions (tension, disgust), shift your attention to another part of the body for a moment. If you still feel uncomfortable, close the magazine and use the relaxation technique, concentrating especially on your breathing.

As you begin to pay more attention to the breasts and genitals in the pictures, start to make some personal observations about their details and to note differences among them. Note, for instance, that some women have more pubic hair than others and how the hair pattern varies from woman to woman. Notice how the skin color and texture varies slightly, too. Does it seem coarse, or smooth and soft? What do you imagine this hair would smell like?

As you look more closely at the pictures of the genitals, notice differences in the thickness of the outer lips of the vagina, as well as their folds and coloring. What do you imagine they would feel like if you touched them, ever so lightly, using the very tips of your fingers?

Notice details about, and differences among, women's breasts, as well as their genitals. See how their size and shape can vary and how different the nipples can be in size, color, and texture. Imagine yourself licking the nipples—what would they feel and taste like?

Continue with this second step until you are able to look at the genitals and breasts in the photos without getting very tense. Then buy yourself a third set of magazines and repeat the looking procedure. Again, it is fine if you become sexually aroused by the photos. In fact, you should repeat buying sets of magazines and looking at the women in detail, especially the breasts and genitals, until you *do* find them to be a turn-on. At that point, you should masturbate, using the photos as stimulation. If you like, make up a fantasy about the women in the pictures and put yourself in the fantasy with them. Or just look at the pictures and get turned on by them. See if you can get turned on by looking at the breasts and genitals, as well as other parts of the bodies.

When you are able to use such photos as a source of stimulation for masturbation and to get turned on by thinking of or looking at the women's breasts and genitals, as well as the rest of their bodies, you are ready to move on to the next exercise. That does not mean, however, that you will no longer have a use for the magazines or that you won't want to buy more from time to time. On the contrary, the more you are able to continue doing the sorts of things described in this exercise, the more likely it is that you will, in time, become increasingly comfortable with real female genitals.

As the next step in the desensitization procedure, you will make use of your own imagination to overcome your discomfort about the female body. Once more the relaxation technique will come in handy, so be sure you have learned it well by now.

Exercise 7.4: Using Your Imagination 1

In this exercise, you will follow along, using your imagination, as you are led through a scene or fantasy. At several points you will be asked to stop imagining the scene and to focus instead on your own body and how it feels. If and when you find yourself feeling tense, you should use the relaxation technique (tense yourself even more just a little, think the word RELAX, let the tension go) before proceeding further.

If you can record the following material, it will increase the effectiveness of the guided fantasy technique over and above what reading it will do for you. If you do decide to record the fantasy, make sure that you speak slowly and clearly. In addition, stop talking, but leave the tape running, for as long as the instructions tell you to (for example: **Pause 30 seconds**). This will create short periods of silence on the tape that you will use for checking out your feelings. It may require several "takes" for you to come up with a good tape recording, but it is worth the time and effort.

You should do this exercise in bed. It will take twenty minutes to half-an-hour, so make sure that you have at least that much uninterrupted privacy. If you have recorded the fantasy, place the recorder close at hand where you can start and stop it whenever you need to without having to get up.

GUIDED FANTASY 1

1 Imagine that you and one of the women from the men's magazines you looked through—a woman you find especially attractive—are sitting at opposite ends of a large, warm, and comfortable bed. The bed is in the middle of a nicely decorated, spacious room with flowered wallpaper and blue curtains. Imagine this setting. See the wallpaper and the curtains.

The room you are in is lighted, but not too brightly, and the air is fresh and sweet smelling. The bed is soft and covered with a gold satin sheet. Imagine how comfortable it is to sit there and imagine the woman being there with you. You are both naked, but she is sitting some distance away, with her back to you. Look at her, starting with her hair. Picture if you can its color, thickness, and shape; imagine what it would feel like and smell like. Look slowly from her hair downward to her neck. Picture her neck. Notice its shape, the color and texture of the skin, its softness and smoothness. See a strand of hair dangling across it, and imagine what it would be like to touch her neck, very lightly, with the tips of your fingers. Breathe in, and imagine how her skin would smell. If you were to lick her there, how would she taste?

Focus for a moment on the base of the woman's neck, where it joins the shoulders. Let your eyes follow this curve, out to one shoulder, then back again. Look at the bottom of her neck, and notice that the skin there is covered with fine, downy hair, delicate and soft. Breathe deeply again, and catch the aroma of her perfume. Let your eyes wander until they find the dimple of her spine, at the top of her back near her neck, and then let your eyes just sort of drift down it, slowly, lazily, down along the smooth soft curve of her spine, until you are looking at her behind. Picture the soft, round curves of her cheeks. Imagine how they would feel if you could reach out and touch them.

   (Pause 15 seconds.)

Notice now how your body feels, by paying attention to different parts of it in turn. If you discover that you are feeling tense, stop your tape recorder and use the relaxation technique. Pay special attention to your breathing. When you feel relaxed again, return to point 1. If you don't seem tense, but are either relaxed or a little turned on, start your recorder again and continue.

   (Pause 10 seconds.)

2 *Imagine the room again and the woman sitting across the bed from you. See her neck, with its fine covering of downy hair. Now let your eyes drift out, following the curve of her shoulder. Follow it around the shoulder and down along the outside of her arm. Notice how much detail you are able to see—the texture and color of the skin tiny, soft hairs freckles or beauty marks. Note how smooth the skin of the upper arm is, then pause to compare it to the skin on the elbow. Look closely and take your time.*

Moving slowly downward once more, see the skin on the woman's forearm, its color and texture. It has a heavier coat of fine, soft hair, and it is slender and delicate in shape. What would it feel like? Smell like? Taste like? Now see her wrist. Notice that it is small and thin. Then see her hand. Follow the wrist to the hand, to the fingers; follow each one of the fingers to the nail. Take it all in and see how attractive it all is. Her nails are long, slender, and painted. Go slowly across her hand, taking the time to notice details, like the color and texture of the skin, its lines and creases. Make a note of the shape of the hand and of each finger. How does the skin on the hand compare to the skin on the forearm, the elbow, the upper arm, and the neck? How would each of these places feel? Would they be the same temperature or different temperatures?

Leaving the one hand now, let your eyes wander across to the woman's back again. Look at it closely. See its shape, its contours and curves, the color and texture of the skin. What would it taste like, do you think? If you could press your face close, what would it smell like?

Let your eyes continue to drift, lazily, downward until they settle once again on her behind. Look at her. Breathe in the smell of her perfume.

(Pause 15 seconds.)

Do a second body check. If you find yourself feeling tense, stop your recorder and use the relaxation technique, then return to point 2. If you feel relaxed, or if this part of the fantasy is getting you turned on, start your recorder again and continue.

(Pause 10 seconds.)

3 *Imagine now that the woman slowly, very slowly, begins to move, turning ever so slowly to face you. She is sitting with her legs crossed and is turning slowly, slowly, as if by magic. See her in profile now, her eyes closed, the curve of a smile on her lips. See her face, following the curve of her profile across her forehead, down along her nose, lips, and chin. See her eyebrows and notice the color of her lips. Focus in on the skin on her cheeks, and imagine how it would feel if you stroked it lightly, gently, using the backs of your fingers. See her eyelashes, long and curved, and see them flutter just the tiniest bit. Then see her lips again. They are full, slightly parted now, slightly moist. The woman smiles, and you see her teeth, white and wet. Look closely at her teeth as she sits across from you, smiling, feeling good.*

Let your eyes slide away from her face, down along her slender neck, down to the upward slope of her breasts. Watch her breasts as she begins to move again, very slowly turning toward you. Note their size and shape. Imagine how they would feel if you stroked them lightly or took them in your hands and squeezed them. See the nipples, their shape, size, color, and texture. How would the nipples feel if you touched them with your fingers? How would they feel if you touched them with your tongue? Imagine the breasts in front of you and see them seem to swell and shrink as the woman breathes.

(Pause 15 seconds.)

Notice how your body is feeling right now. If you seem tense, stop the tape, relax yourself, and then return to point 3. Otherwise proceed with the fantasy.

(Pause 10 seconds.)

4 *Imagine now that the woman has turned completely around and is facing you. Look at her breasts again. They are full, but not too large; they are round, smooth, and soft looking. Lift your eyes and find yourself looking into hers. Give her eyes color and shape; imagine them made up if you like. Imagine yourself sitting there, looking into her eyes, and see her begin to smile again,* slightly at first, and gradually more and more. Let yourself smile back. Take a deep breath and hear and see her do the same. Smell her.

Her face is pretty and very sensual. You can feel your sexual attraction to her. It is a force inside of you that she sets loose. Watch her eyes now as they begin to wander across your own body. See her look at your shoulders and then at your chest, your stomach, genitals, and legs. She looks at your penis again, this time pausing to stare at it for a moment. She smiles again into your eyes.

Now her eyes wander, as you watch them, across your shoulders, down your arms, along your hands. And as she sits there taking you in, your own eyes wander away from hers and drift slowly down to her breasts, then past her breasts to her stomach. Imagine the way her stomach looks. See the navel, its size and shape, and the soft textures of the skin around it. Do you see any hair or is it perfectly smooth and hairless? What would it feel like to touch her stomach with your wrist? What would its temperature be, warm or cool?

Your eyes drift downward again, slowly and patiently making their way from the stomach to the very top of the genital area, stopping at the spot where the pubic hair begins, which you can just make out above the tops of her crossed legs. Let yourself look at this for a moment, more carefully and closely than you ever have before.

(Pause 15 seconds.)

Notice the way your body is responding to the fantasy now. If you are tense, stop the tape and relax yourself, then return to point 4. If you feel either relaxed or sexually excited, proceed with the fantasy.

(Pause 10 seconds.)

5 Imagine that the woman has closed her eyes again. She looks happy, comfortable, and content as she sits in front of you. She sighs. See her chest move, hear her breathe. Let yourself breathe in the aroma of her perfume, mixed with the natural aroma of her body.

While she sits there with her eyes closed, take your time and notice in detail the way her genital hair looks. See its color, density, and pattern. What does the skin beneath it look like? If you were to take some of the hair and rub it between your thumb and forefinger, what would it feel like?

Imagine now that, as you stare into her genital area, the woman slowly, ever so slowly, begins to uncross her legs. Very slowly they unlock and begin to spread apart. Watch it happening.

As the woman's legs slowly spread apart, her thighs and genitals gradually come into view, dimly at first, in shadow, but then, slowly, more clearly. Imagine now that she leans back on her arms, her legs spread wide before you. Her eyes are still closed, a comfortable, happy smile on her lips. She is sitting just beyond your reach, but you can smell the aroma of her body now, not perfumed, but still sweet, and you can hear her breathing, even and deep. Now you can also see her thighs and genitals quite clearly. You glance at them and then look up at her content expression. She likes you to look at her—to appreciate her body. She sighs again, and then opens her eyes and looks at you. See her smile grow wider. You smile back and see her look now at her own genitals. Let your eyes follow her lead. See her thighs, soft, smooth, and appealing. Follow them inward, toward her genitals. See the hair again and then the lips of her vagina.

(Pause 15 seconds.)

Do another body check and, if you are tense, stop the tape and relax yourself, then go back to point 5. Otherwise continue with the fantasy.

(Pause 10 seconds.)

6 *Let your attention come to rest now on the woman's genitals. Let your eyes wander from place to place. Notice details that you never noticed before. Take your time, keeping in mind that the woman likes to be looked at in this way—as a sexual, physically attractive being.*

What do the outer lips of the vagina look like, now that you can take your time and look at them clearly? What is their color? What would they feel like? Imagine that they would smell, not like perfume, but sweet and natural. And what do you imagine they might taste like and feel like if you touched them with your tongue? Would they be cold or warm, warmer than any other part of her, and soft as velvet?

(Pause 15 seconds.)

Do a final body check. If the last part of the fantasy made you tense, stop the tape, pause to relax, and then try again from point 6. If you feel relaxed or sexually excited, stop the tape and lie back for a while, concentrating on taking deep, easy breaths.

Exercise 7.4 should be done completely several times before you attempt to move on. Your goal is to be able to complete the guided fantasy, making it as real as possible in your imagination, without getting tense or anxious. This may not be possible the first time you try the exercise. It is important to the desensitization procedure, however, that you move ahead *only* when your anxiety at one step has been reduced or replaced by feelings of sexual arousal. For this reason it is important that you proceed only as directed, which is to say that you stop and back up a bit whenever you sense yourself getting tense.

It is fine, of course, if you experience feelings of sexual arousal when you go through the guided fantasy, but you should still move only as fast as the instructions direct you. That is, don't skip exercises or move through any one of them too fast. If you are not yet experiencing any sexual arousal, don't be too concerned. Before sexual excitement can occur, you need to overcome the anxiety that is associated with your genital phobia. It will be very important for you to keep in mind, as you proceed, that physical signs of slight sexual arousal can at times feel like signs of discomfort or anxiety, so do not confuse the two.

In Exercise 7.4, you focused your imagination on the problem of discomfort with women's bodies. This technique of using a guided fantasy to bring you, through your imagination, in contact with what makes you uncomfortable is one way to help desensitize you to your discomfort. The following exercise is a continuation of this same process.

Exercise 7.5: Using Your Imagination 2

Again, if possible, record the guided fantasy described below and play it back to yourself, rather than simply reading it to yourself. Be sure to read into the recorder slowly and clearly and to pause whenever the instructions call for it. Do the exercise in bed when you will have at least half-an-hour.

Lie back, relax, and imagine the following scene as vividly as possible.

GUIDED FANTASY 2

1 *You and one of the women from the magazine photos (you can picture the same woman or make up a different woman from the one in Exercise 7.4) are naked together in a bathroom. It is a large room, comfortable, clean, and warm. It has walls painted in a soft yellow and a large, shaggy white rug. You and the woman are standing close together, but not touching, on this rug. You look at each other and smile. Imagine yourself looking at the woman's naked body as she stands in front of you. See her face, her hair, her neck, her shoulders, and her arms. Now picture her breasts, her stomach, and her genitals. See her thighs, her legs, and her feet. She is extremely attractive and very happy to be there with you. Look at her and see her smile at you. Smile back at her and hear yourself telling her how beautiful her body is and how much you enjoy looking at it.*

(**Pause 15 seconds.**)

Shift your attention to your own inner feelings now and do a body check. If you find that you are tense, stop the tape, pause, and relax yourself. Then return to point 1. If you feel relaxed, or even a little turned on, proceed with the fantasy.

(**Pause 10 seconds.**)

2 *Imagine now that the woman begins to look at your body as you stand before her. Imagine her looking at your face, your neck, your shoulders, and arms. Watch her eyes as she looks at* *your chest, your stomach, and now your genitals. See her looking at your penis and smiling. Feel how good she makes you feel. See her looking at your thighs, your legs, and your feet. She looks up at you, catches your eye, and smiles again. Hear her tell you how much she likes your body, and feel yourself respond to her. She makes you feel warm and comfortable, and maybe a little excited. You look at her, up and down, and marvel at how beautiful her body is, all of it.*

Watch now as the woman turns. Gracefully, she leaves the rug and steps over to a large tub. She reaches out and draws the curtain aside. With a glance over her shoulder at you, she enters the tub and lets the curtain fall closed behind her. A moment later you hear the sound of the water being turned on. Hear the sound of it hitting the bottom of the tub and the curtain. Hear the woman sigh as the warm water begins to wash over her body.

A moment later, a hand appears at the edge of the curtain. It moves back. Then she peeks at you, smiling, and winks. You smile back. She gives you a nod, and you go to her. She holds the curtain back for you.

You are together again, standing close to one another, but still not touching. You are close enough to smell her clearly and to hear the sounds of her breathing. See her chest heave, her nostrils flare, as she sighs beneath the spray, turning her face upward in obvious pleasure. See her standing beneath the spray, directly under the nozzle, her eyes closed, moving her head so that the clean warm water can soak her hair, her face, her neck, and ears. See the water splashing against her face, her neck, and her shoulders; see her skin glisten. She smiles.

Now, as you watch, she begins to turn slowly around. Once, then twice she turns completely around, so that the water can wash over all of her. Look at each part of her in turn as the water sprays against her body; her shoulders, back, and breasts; her stomach and behind; her genitals, her thighs, legs, and feet. Watch her body closely, paying attention to details as she displays herself in front of you. She is enjoying the water, and she is enjoying your looking at her. See the way her skin sparkles and how clean and smooth she looks. Think about how it would feel if you were the water, running across her body. Now see her stop and open her eyes. Feel your eyes meet, staring at each other across the narrow space between you.

(Pause 15 seconds.)

Notice how your body feels at this moment. If you are tense, stop the tape, relax for a moment or two, and then return to point 2. Otherwise proceed.

(Pause 10 seconds.)

3 *See the woman again, standing in front of you in the shower. The spray is hitting against her shoulders, sending off drops that land on your face and chest. Feel them as they hit you. See her extend a hand toward you, your own reaching out to meet it. Feel your hands touching, hers squeezing yours ever so lightly. Feel the tug of her pull. You move forward, toward her. Feel the water begin to hit you more directly now, first against your chest, then on your face and shoulders. Feel your hand being squeezed lightly again. Feel her hand—warm and delicate. She moves your hand toward her face, placing your fingers against her cheek. Look closely at her face, into her eyes. Notice the color and texture of her complexion. She is very pretty, and she obviously likes you. Imagine yourself gently stroking her cheek, feeling its warm wetness. See her close her eyes and smile; hear her sigh in response to your touch.*

Move your hand slowly from her cheek down to her neck. Softly run your fingers along the sides of her neck, feeling its smoothness. Use the very tips of your fingers to sense its softness, and then make your way gradually across to her shoulder. Feel its curve and the skin beneath your touch. Picture its color. Now imagine that she lazily lifts her arms over her head and closes her eyes. See her underarms and focus your attention on them as she turns slowly around, smiling all the while, letting the warm spray massage her body. Your hand reaches out and touches her beneath the arm, then strokes her very gently. She sighs.

(Pause 15 seconds.)

Shift once more to your own body and note your feelings. If you feel relaxed, or sexually aroused, continue; but if you are tense, stop the tape, pause to relax yourself, and then return to point 3.

(Pause 10 seconds.)

4 *Look now at the woman's breasts. Notice their size and shape and how smooth the skin is. See how they move as she breathes. Imagine the water running across them, first one, then the other. Watch it wash over the nipples and see her close her eyes and smile at the pleasant feelings this gives her.*

Now feel yourself reaching out to touch her breasts. See yourself touching one of them, very lightly, then more firmly. Feel its softness through your finger tips. Press lightly against it. Feel the warmth of the water running over and around them. Stroke the breast, once, twice, three times. See the woman close her eyes; hear her sigh at the good feelings you give her. Continue stroking it lightly and watch as the nipple changes shape, becoming firmer, more erect. Take the erect nipple between your thumb and forefinger and rub it lightly. Hear the woman sigh and see her body move in response.

Now take her whole breast into your hand, cupping it in your palm. Squeeze it very lightly at first, then harder. Rub it in your palm and at the same time imagine that the woman opens her eyes and looks at you. You continue stroking her breast, and she smiles. Hear yourself tell her how good her breast feels to you and how good you feel when you look at her.

(Pause 15 seconds.)

Check to see how you are feeling right now. Stop the tape to pause and relax if you feel tense, then return to point 4. If you're feeling good—relaxed or turned on—proceed with the fantasy.

(Pause 10 seconds.)

5 *See yourself moving closer now. Feel your legs move. As you approach her, see the woman slowly turn, so that by the* time you are close enough to touch she has turned her back to you. You are standing so close that your bodies can touch each other with the slightest movement, but you are not touching yet. Imagine how it feels to be this close, yet not to touch. You want to touch and she wants to be touched.

The spray from the shower washes over both of you now equally. It hits her shoulders, your chest, running down her back, your front. See yourself reaching out to touch her back. See the clean, glistening skin before you and feel it through your fingers. It is exciting to touch her now, to feel her warm body, and experience her response to your hand. Let your fingers run up and down her back, then again, using a firmer touch. Hear and feel her sigh beneath your touch. Notice how smooth she is, how warm and clean. Tell her how good her body looks and how exciting it is to touch her.

Imagine that your hand gradually wanders downward, from her back to her waist, pausing there to take in the sensation of its curves, and then down to her cheeks. You run your fingers across them, first one, then the other. Feel how soft and smooth she is there as you stroke her, up and down, side to side, in straight lines, and then in circles. Hear her sigh again. Look down at her behind. It is smooth, clean, and attractive. Like the rest of her, it glistens beneath the warm water.

Touch the small of her back now. Even with the water running across it, you can feel, through the very tips of your fingers, the fine, downy hairs that cover it. From there your fingers slip, very easily, without effort or thought, into the space between her cheeks. They wander across it, exploring its texture. Passing over the dimple of her anus, they make the woman sigh yet again, so you press one finger into it, lightly, not enough to penetrate but enough to give her pleasure. Then you run your hand up and down along her crack, using lighter, then heavier pressure, noting the way she reacts to this. Experience the pleasure you can give through your hand.

Now the woman, clearly feeling excited by your touch, begins to turn toward you, and as she does your hand slips out from her.

You look at each other, and she tells you, not through words so much as the look in her eyes, how much you please her.

(Pause 15 seconds.)

Do a body check. Once again, tension is your cue to stop the tape, relax, and then back up to point 5. Otherwise you may proceed.

(Pause 10 seconds.)

6 *You are still looking at each other, and now your bodies are touching. She is breathing heavily, obviously turned on by your touch. She reaches out with both hands and takes your face. Feel her touch against your cheeks. Feel her warmth and caring, expressed now in the way she strokes you. From your cheeks her fingers wander down to your neck, then across your shoulders and down your arms. Your own body, like hers, is warm. It, too, is clean and glistens beneath the water. Feel her fingers as they run down your arms, caressing them. Feel your lungs fill as you sigh. The way she touches you makes you feel so good that you cannot keep your eyes open, so you close them and imagine her touching you as you feel it happening. You can hear her breathing; you can smell her; and your awareness of her hands on your body is so very clear to you. Your own breathing, in response to her, gradually becomes deeper, heavier, and marked by sighs. She presses her fingers into your armpits, and as she does your arms loosen completely, relaxed. She strokes your sides, up and down, up and down, lightly at first, now pressing harder. Then she is at your waist. She strokes you lightly again, then presses her body up against yours. Feel her against you, so close, and feel her hands working their way across your back. Her fingernails tease you, and you respond with a sign; they dig into your flesh, not too hard, but enough to draw a groan of pleasure from deep inside you.*

Now she backs away from you, and as she does, you feel her hands again, on your stomach, moving downward. Her nails scratch your pubic hair, then rub it lightly. A moment later her gentle hands are gliding across your genitals, stroking your penis. She takes the head between her fingers and rubs it. Imagine the sensations that this gives you, not only in your penis, but all through your body. It is as though your nerves went from it to everywhere in you. Then she caresses your scrotum, taking you into both her hands at once. Hear yourself sigh, then her. Open your eyes and find her looking at you with great passion.

(Pause 15 seconds.)

How do you feel right now? Tense? If so, stop the tape, relax, then back up to point 6. Otherwise proceed.

(Pause 10 seconds.)

7 *Imagine yourself telling the woman how good her touch feels, how much you enjoy being touched. And now imagine yourself reaching out yet again, this time touching her stomach. It feels warm, soft, and smooth. You let a finger slip into her navel, twisting it gently. You tell her once more how nice her body is and how much you enjoy touching it and looking at it. She smiles and tells you that you give her a lot of pleasure.*

Let your hand glide along her body, from her stomach to her genitals. Run your fingers lightly through her pubic hair, and as you do, look down at her genitals. See her hair, its color, its thickness. See it move as the water washes through it. Feel its soft wetness through your fingers.

Press the palm of your hand into her, so that the whole of her genitals are in it. Feel its warmth. You look down at your hand, touching her, and then up into her eyes. She smiles at you. Gently, you rub your palm against her genitals and watch her response. First she sighs, her eyes closing. Then she moans, her face turning upward. Through your hand you feel her body shiver. Then, as you continue to rub her with your palm, her breathing deepens, becomes heavier. After a while, her body begins to tremble and she begins to moan with each breath. She reaches out and puts her arms around you, pulling you close, holding you. You stop your rubbing, but leave your hand still cradling her genitals. The water is still running across them and your hand. It feels warm and soothing, and you just stand there for a moment, holding her close to you, feeling her through the palm of your hand.

After holding her for a little while, your hand again begins to move. Instead of your palm, your fingers now explore her. You touch the outer lips of her vagina, tracing them from top to bottom, then back again. They are soft, like velvet. As you explore them, using the very tips of your fingers, watch her reaction. See, feel, and hear her begin to get excited again in response to you.

You run your fingers lightly along the slit between the outer lips, and then, easily, you slide one finger between the folds. Imagine penetrating her with just one finger, just up to the first knuckle, and feel the insides of the lips. Notice the texture of the skin, its delicacy and softness. As you move your finger deeper, just a little, you come to the inner lips and then to the opening to the vagina itself, with the very tip of your finger. Feel how soft it is, how warm, and moist. Push again, gently, and feel your finger penetrating the vagina, moving easily because of the moist lubrication of sexual arousal. Feel the walls of the vagina and feel them press back against your finger, enclosing and holding it. Then, as the muscles behind the vagina contract, feel it squeeze you gently for a moment. As this happens, notice the way the walls of the vagina feel, smooth and just the slightest bit rippled. Slide your finger in and out slowly several times, and then twist it from side to side. Experience the sensations of containment—containment made comfortable by the warm lubricating fluid and the smooth vaginal lining. Experience again the way in which the vagina can hold you and the way your partner can squeeze you, when she wishes, by flexing her muscles.

See yourself looking down now. See your own finger, inserted into the woman's vagina, and watch it emerge as you slowly pull it out. See how moist and clean it is. Look up at the woman again, meet her eyes, and smile.

(Pause 15 seconds.)

How are you feeling? If the final part of the fantasy made you tense, pause to relax, and then return to point 7. Otherwise you are finished with the fantasy.

Exercise 7.5 should be done several times. As in the previous exercise, it may take a while for you to be able to complete it without becoming tense. Let your tension be your guide. Take it as a sign that you need to pause, relax yourself, and back up a step. Once you are able to get through this second guided fantasy without becoming tense, it is very likely that you will begin to experience feelings of sexual arousal. In fact, this can happen the very first time you go through the fantasy. These feelings may not be very intense at first, and so you might mistake them for feelings of discomfort. Try to avoid making this mistake. After a while, your feelings of arousal should become strong enough that you won't mistake them for something else. When this begins to happen, you may move on to the next step in the desensitization procedure, described below.

If you are now at the point where you are able to complete Exercise 7.5 without anxiety, perhaps even experiencing some sexual arousal, your genital phobia should be much improved. You may be able to improve it further by asking your partner to allow you to explore her body, much the way Exercise 7.5 had you explore a woman's body in fantasy. If you think she might be willing, ask your partner to read the following exercise and give it some thought. Then decide together if you want to go through with it.

Exercise 7.6: Exploring Bodies

Begin the exercise by both taking showers. If you prefer, you can take separate showers, but consider doing it together. If this is something you haven't done before, try it as an experiment. It can be a lot of fun, if you let it be.

In the shower, take turns soaping one another all over, including genitals. Do this gently, playfully—don't try to scrub each other down. Take your time and talk to each other. Say how it feels to wash the other person and how it feels to be washed by someone else. Then take a minute to show each other how you wash yourselves when you take showers alone.

After the shower, take turns drying each other, including genitals. Be gentle, not rough. Then sprinkle some powder over each other and rub it in. Do the shoulders, backs, chests, arms, and legs. Don't pour on the powder, but just sprinkle it lightly. After you are finished, go to the bedroom or some other private place together. Make sure that this place was prepared in advance, that it is comfortable, warm enough, and lighted (but not too brightly). Also make sure that you will not be interrupted for at least one hour.

> *Ask your partner to lie down on her stomach while you sit or kneel beside her. Using a light, gentle touch, start to explore her body. If at any time during this process of exploration, you find yourself feeling tense, pause for a moment, use the relaxation technique, and then return to what you were doing. If you still feel anxious, try relaxing again, and then shift your attention and explore a different part of the body than the one you were touching when you became tense.*
>
> *Begin your exploration at your partner's head. Touch her hair, noticing closely its color and texture. Is it the same color all over, or does the color vary? Lightly massage the scalp and note the way your partner's head feels when you touch it this way.*
>
> *Move from your partner's head to her neck and shoulders. Use light, gentle strokes and tune in to the feelings in your sensitive finger tips, to experience the textures of your partner's body. Look for differences in smoothness, temperature, and softness. Look closely at skin color and take in the aroma of her body. Try to open all your senses and take in as much as you can. Practice sexual communication skills by letting your partner know it if you like the way some part of her feels, smells, or looks. To experience the pleasure you are capable of giving with your hands, pay attention now and then to your partner's nonverbal reactions—sighs, moans, and movements. Try to discover something about the kinds of touching that please her most.*

Make your way slowly down from the neck and shoulders to your partner's back. Use your finger tips, your palms, and the insides of your wrists to experience how her body feels. Stroke lightly, then more firmly. Notice how her skin feels different, depending on what part of you is touching her; fingers versus palms, fingers versus wrists, and so on. Look closely at the color of the skin, then bend down close enough to sniff it. Run your hands up and down in long stroking movements and feel its curves and contours. When you feel ready to leave it, move from the back down to the buttocks. Before you do, however, pay some attention to your own body and how you are feeling. If you feel good—relaxed or sexually turned on—say something about that to your partner. If you are feeling tense, let her know that, too, and then follow the same instructions—pause, relax yourself, and try again.

Spend some time now exploring your partner's lower back and buttocks. Feel how soft the skin is in the small of the back. Look closely and see if you can see fine, downy hairs. Touch them and watch your partner's reactions. Move down and begin to stroke your partner's behind. Stroke one cheek, then the other, very lightly, then more firmly. Note your partner's reactions to these different sorts of touch. Then run your fingers along the crevice between her cheeks, and then press them into it. Run your fingers along her crack and press one finger against the anus, firmly but not hard enough to penetrate. Notice the reaction you get. Then run your fingers up and down once more, along the crack, until you come in contact with the beginning of your partner's genitals, and then take your hand away.

Leave the buttocks for now and move downward again, to the thighs. Stroke them all over, using different pressures. Again, use your fingers, your palms, and your wrists. Bend down to smell the skin and use your tongue to taste it (and as something else to feel with as well). Look closely at the skin. Is its texture the same on the inside of the thighs as on the outside? Is it different from, or the same as, the skin on her back? What sorts of reactions does your touching bring out, and what kind of touching does your partner seem to enjoy most?

Work your way slowly from the thighs, to the legs, to the feet. Pay attention to the skin on your partner's legs. Take a calf in both hands and squeeze it to feel the muscles beneath. Stroke it lightly to experience its shape and texture. Notice the reactions you get. Smell it; taste it if you like.

Move yourself so that you can get to your partner's feet without having to bend too far. Look at them. Notice the way the skin is different on different parts of the feet, thicker and thinner, rougher and smoother. Touch the sides and then the soles, again noticing the differences. Does your partner seem very sensitive to touch on her feet, and if so, where does she seem to be most sensitive?

Pause for a moment. Stop touching your partner, sit still, and close your eyes. Take several deep breaths. When you feel relaxed and ready to continue, ask your partner to roll over onto her back and begin to explore her once more. Sit by her head again and begin your exploring with her face. Look at it as you touch it. Use the tips of your fingers to explore its contours and textures. Touch her forehead, her eyebrows, her ears, nose, lips, and chin. Stroke her cheeks. If something feels or looks good to you, tell her so. Moving at your own pace, but not hurrying in any way, make your way down along her neck to her shoulders, then across her soulders to her arms. Do each arm separately, looking at it closely. Move each one away from her body so that you can look at and touch her underarms. Let your hand rest there and feel its warmth. If your partner has hair beneath her arms, note its color, its length, and its texture. Take some between your thumb and forefinger and smell it. Then move down the arms, one at a time. Touch each upper arm, each elbow, each forearm. Pay attention to skin color and texture and to differences, for example, between the upper arm and forearm and the insides and outsides of the forearms. Look at your partner's hair—its color, fineness, and thickness. Stroke it lightly and watch the reaction you get. People's bodies really are very sensitive in so very many places, and there is so much that they are capable of giving to and receiving from one another if they want to give and take.

228 BECOMING SATISFIED

Now look at each one of your partner's hands very closely. Touch them all over. Take your time. Touch each one of the fingers; stroke lightly in between the fingers. Massage each one for a moment or two and see how pleasing this can be to your partner.

When you feel ready to leave your partner's hands, move on to her breasts. First, just look at them. Look at them more closely than you have before. Take your time. Notice their size, their shape. Watch them move as your partner breathes. Look at the nipples—their color and shape, as well as their texture. Now touch one breast, using your finger tips. Explore it for a while, paying attention not so much to your partner's reactions as to the way her breast feels to you. Then stroke it lightly and notice her responses. Experiment with different kinds of strokes. Look at the nipple again. Has its color changed? Is it erect (firm) now? Cup the breast in your hand and squeeze it, then rub it. How does it feel to you and how does your partner react? Look at the nipple again. Take it between your thumb and forefinger and caress it. Then bend over and lick it lightly, just once or twice. How does it feel through your tongue and how does it taste? Stroke the whole breast again, this time using your wrist. See how this feels to you and, again, how your partner reacts, especially nonverbally. Discover not only something about her body and how it feels to you, but the way she responds and what she seems to like the most. As you do this, don't worry too much if you make a "mistake" (press or squeeze too hard, for instance). Just learn from your exploring and be patient with yourself.

Spend some time exploring your partner's other breast, and then move on to explore her stomach. See how smooth the skin is. Notice any fine hairs. Lay your hand on the stomach and feel its warmth. Stroke it lightly. Smell the skin, taste it, or both.

As you feel ready, move down to your partner's genitals, exploring them briefly. Look at and touch the pubic hair. Run your fingers through it, then take some in your fingers and feel the texture. Smell it. Look at your partner's genitals for a moment, and then move on.

Spend some time exploring the front of your partner's legs. Look at and touch the thighs again. Experiment with different strokes and different amounts of pressure. Use different parts of you to touch with. Do this with the calves as well, and then work your way gradually to the feet. Notice how soft the skin is on the top of the feet. Run your fingers across the toes and then massage them. Finally, experiment with stroking in between the toes. Notice the way your partner responds to you.

Slowly, make your way back up toward your partner's genitals. Look at them and then look at the rest of her. Try to think of the genitals as one part of a whole person, as something connected to a person, rather than something foreign or apart. When you feel ready, reach out and run your fingers through the pubic hair again. From there let your fingers slowly, comfortably work their way downward into your partner's crotch. Follow the contours of the skin, and watch your own hand as it does so. Look at the outer lips of the vagina, and use your sensitive finger tips to explore them. Take your time, don't hurry. Use a very light touch at first, and then a slightly heavier touch. Use heavier touches until you finally use enough pressure so that your finger slips into the crevice formed by the outer lips. Then, very slowly, move your finger up and down. Feel the warmth and texture of this interior skin. Is it moist? How does your partner react to your finger moving along the insides of her lips?

Now let your fingers follow the crevice upward to the point at which the lips join. This is where your partner's clitoris is. The clitoris, like the head of your penis, is very sensitive, and clitoral stimulation is generally necessary for orgasm in women, just as stimulation of the head of your penis is necessary for you to reach orgasm. Stroke the skin around the clitoris (that is, in the area around where the lips come together) very lightly a few times, and note your partner's response. Notice, using your finger tips, the firmness of the clitoral area. See if you can detect the small, roundish form of the clitoris itself beneath its hood of skin. As your partner becomes sexually aroused, the clitoris, like her nipples, becomes firmer and a little larger than it otherwise is. See if you can detect this happening now, as you continue your light stroking in that area. Then try to discover, by using different amounts of pressure and stroking in different places and different ways, the kind(s) of clitoral stimulation your partner likes best. Don't, however, go so far as to bring her to orgasm—yet.

Now guide your fingers down along the outer lips again. If your partner's legs are together, open them. Using only slight pressure, slip one of your fingers between the outer lips again. Penetrate far enough so that you can just feel the entrance to the vagina with your finger tip. Pause for a moment there and notice the sensations in your finger, the pressure, the temperature, the moistness. Now, penetrate farther, moving slowly into the vagina itself. Note your partner's reaction to this. Push your finger in as far as you (and your partner) feel comfortable doing, and then be still. Look at your partner's genitals while you focus on the sensations in your finger. Feel how the vagina accommodates it, snugly but not too tightly. The vagina is capable of expanding and contracting, so that it can hold a penis in just this very way. Press your finger against the wall of the vagina, but not so hard that your partner feels uncomfortable. Ask her if she can flex the muscles behind her vagina to squeeze your finger. Then be still again. Feel the warmth of the vagina.

Now, if and only if your partner wants you to, try moving your finger in and out of her vagina, imitating the motion of intercourse. Notice her response, but notice also the sensations in your finger as it moves. Notice how well the vaginal lubrication that your partner's body produces works to make the movements smooth and easy. Feel the light pressure of the vagina against your finger. When a larger object, such as your penis, is inserted in place of your finger, the vagina will expand in such a way as to maintain just about this same amount of pressure.

If your explorations have gotten your partner turned on, you should feel free now to satisfy her in any way you like. Exploring may also have gotten you excited, and lovemaking may be the best prescription for the two of you. Go ahead.

Once you have completed an exploration of your partner's body, and perhaps made love, it would be a good idea if you could change places. Lie down on your stomach and let her begin to explore your body. Let her take as much time as she likes. You will probably find this every bit as enjoyable as she does.

It would be good if you could do Exercise 7.6 more than once. Each time you may discover new things about each others' bodies that can add much to your sexual relationship in the future. Your minimum goal is to be able to do the exercise without feeling anxious. Depending on the severity of your discomfort with the female body, this may take one, two, or many attempts. If, after a while, you begin to find the exercise sexually arousing (or if you do from the first), that is even better. However, you should not necessarily expect your discomfort to disappear quickly or suddenly; more likely there will be a gradual improvement. Even if you do enjoy the exercise as a whole, you may not feel comfortable exploring your partner's genitals the first few times you try it. Most likely you will experience a steady, slow decline in your level of discomfort, followed by an equally steady rise in your level of sexual excitement. Try not to mistake these early signs of slight arousal for feelings of discomfort.

SUMMARY

This chapter is aimed at helping men who are uncomfortable with women to overcome their discomfort. One type of discomfort is called sexual shyness. It has to do with avoiding women socially, or at least sexually, because of negative expectations about what will happen. For men who experience sexual shyness, starting (or restarting) their social life is the goal to achieve by moving in a step-by-step manner. The relaxation technique can aid in moving yourself in that direction.

For men whose avoidance of women has to do with previous sexual difficulties, and consequently a fear of failing, the key to overcoming their discomfort really has to do mainly with reassessing their attitudes toward themselves. Realizing that men are not sexual machines and that it really is okay for your sexual performance to vary will go a long way toward relieving worries about getting close. Besides this, some plain old motivation is necessary to push yourself into situations that make you nervous, in order to deal with them. When you do get to a place where sexual contact is a possibility, two options are open—you can express your fears to a woman in advance of any sexual contact between you or you can take a chance, have a sexual encounter, and enjoy yourselves even if your penis does not act exactly as you would like it to.

The second form of discomfort about women is more specific than the first. Sexual phobia refers to feelings of discomfort about women's bodies. Many men have mild sexual phobias, but some experience such extreme reactions that it ruins their sexual relationships or causes them to avoid women. At times this sort of discomfort may be realistic—concerning something about a particular woman's body—but more often it is a general uneasiness about bodies that stems from upbringing and the sexual attitudes developed as a child. Dealing with this problem involves a procedure known as desensitization. By using the relaxation technique and moving once more in a step-by-step manner, you can in time learn to overcome your inhibitions and not only feel comfortable with your partner's body, but genuinely enjoy it. Needless to say, changes such as these will lead directly to improvements in your social life, your sexual relationship, or both.

8 understanding erection problems

There is probably no sexual dysfunction so distressing to a man as difficulty in getting or maintaining an erection. Even one such experience is usually upsetting, more so for those who believe the old myths about the male as an unfailing sex machine. Of the men I have spoken to or worked with as a sex therapist, those who have experienced these particular sorts of sexual difficulties over a period of time are by far the most uptight and upset. They feel more than embarrassed about their problem; often they feel downright ashamed. It tends, moreover, to affect their entire lives, not just their sexual relationships. Men who were once self-confident and outgoing can become socially withdrawn and depressed. Not only does it become difficult for them to face the possibility of a sexual encounter with a woman, they usually feel weak and inferior in relation to other men as well. Their feelings about their partners tend toward resentment and bitterness. Chronic erection problems can have no less than disastrous effects on marriages.

Given the facts of male sexual anatomy, plus our traditional ideas about male sexuality, it is little wonder that erection problems would elicit such intense reactions and have the potential to be so personally damaging and harmful to relationships. On the purely physical level, intercourse becomes more and more difficult as a man has less and less of an erection. Since intercourse is, after all, a very pleasurable activity from the point of view of the vast majority of men and women, not having an erection, or having one but losing it, is understandably frustrating. This, however, is the least of it. True, an erect penis is important from a purely mechanical standpoint. But erections also have a great deal of *meaning* to both men and women. For one thing, an erect penis has traditionally been taken to be a symbol of sexual desire. That is, an erect penis has been considered to be a sign of a man's sexual interest and of a woman's sexual desirability. Even though a man may feel very sexually attracted, if his penis is not erect, both he and his partner will be inclined to harbor doubts about his interest, her desirability, or both.

The more often it happens that a man's penis does not get (or stay) erect during a sexual encounter, the more likely both partners are to doubt themselves. The woman may feel that she is not sexually attractive, perhaps not skillful enough, or she may come to feel that her partner's "problem" has nothing to do with her, but is a sign of something wrong with him. For his part, the man may blame his partner, thinking that she is not attractive or skillful enough, or he may question his own virility. It is not uncommon for one or both partners to wonder whether a man who experiences such difficulties regularly may be a latent homosexual, but it is more common still for them to think that his problem is a sign that there is something seriously wrong with their relationship. None of these possibilities is necessarily true (there may not be anything seriously wrong with either person or with the relationship), but that is the way people seem to think.

Because an erection is such an important *sign* to him, having many implications about manhood, strength, and so on, a man who experiences erection problems will be tempted to pursue other partners to prove his virility. Since it is also an important sign to a woman about her personal attractiveness, the woman whose partner is experiencing an erection problem will also be tempted to look elsewhere to verify her desirability. It is easy to see the risks involved there; such feelings can wreck a relationship in no time.

For men, the ability to get and keep an erection has also been taken as a sign of personal power, vitality, and strength—hence the term *potency*. A man who can "get it up" feels strong and youthful. The man who has difficulties getting, or keeping, erections not only feels he has a specific sexual problem, but will more than likely also feel weak and inferior to other men. We place so much importance on the ability to get erections, in fact, that a man can easily conclude that his sex life is over if and when he gets to a point where he can't "get it up." He may even feel that his life in general is over. Unfortunately, because they feel so ashamed about it, many men who do experience erection problems of one sort or another put off doing something about them, often for years. During this time they may end their marriages and/or avoid women altogether.

To summarize, the main reasons why erection problems are so embarrassing to men have little to do with the physical significance of an erect penis (as something to use in intercourse), but rather with the meaning and importance our culture has placed on an erection as a *symbol* of sexual desire and personal power. The burden of meaning that an erect penis must bear is heavy and makes erection problems more difficult to deal with than they might otherwise be.

ASSESSING THE PROBLEM

If you have been experiencing erection problems, this book, and even more specifically the program described in this and the following chapter, can help. It will take patience and determination, but you can overcome your sexual dysfunction. If you use this program properly, it may be enough. If it is not enough to overcome the problem, however, there is no reason for you to give up hope. It may be that you need therapy with a trained sex therapist, or it may be a matter of following the program here more consistently; that is, sticking to it better.

As a beginning step in dealing with your erection problem, do the following exercise designed to help you understand your particular problem better.

Exercise 8.1: Pinpointing the Difficulty

When each in a group of men says that he has an erection problem, the individuals are not all talking about the same problem. There are, in other words, different kinds of erection problems. These varieties do not all have the same causes nor are they all treated in exactly the same manner. Getting a clear definition of your problem is important, therefore, for two reasons. First, it will lead to some idea of what you are up against in the way of difficulty. Some erection problems respond to treatment better than others do. Second, a proper diagnosis will serve as a guide to initial treatment.

First, answer each of the questions on the Erection Dysfunction Questionnaire that follows.

ERECTION DYSFUNCTION QUESTIONNAIRE

1. Have you *ever* in your life experienced an erection, through *any* means of stimulation? That is, have you had at least one erection in your life through masturbation, reading, pictures, movies, or by being stimulated by someone else? ____yes ____no
2. Are you *currently* able to experience an erection through at least *one* means of stimulation? ____yes ____no
3. Have you *ever* in your life experienced an erection during a sexual encounter with a woman? ____yes ____no
4. Do you sometimes wake up in the morning and discover that you have an erection? ____yes ____no
5. If you masturbate, do you feel that the erections you get at such times are about as firm and full as they were a year ago? ____yes ____no

6. Can you *sometimes* get either a full or a partial erection during a sexual encounter? ____yes ____no
7. Do you currently experience erections that are full enough for you to have intercourse during at least *some* of your sexual encounters? ____yes ____no
8. Do you have your erection problem with one sexual partner but not another? ____yes ____no
9. Do you feel that you have lost interest in having sex with your usual partner, and that this happened *before* your erection problem began? ____yes ____no

If you answered *no* to question 1, your erection problem is obviously of a fairly severe form. This does *not* necessarily mean that you have an "incurable" condition. However, the fact that you have never experienced an erection at all means that it is important in your case to rule out the possibility that the problem has a physical cause. This requires a thorough physical examination by a licensed medical doctor. Consult your family physician, if you have one; if not, see a physician specializing in urology or internal medicine. Don't put it off and don't assume that a simple, quick checkup will be enough. You need to discuss the sexual problem specifically and explain that you would like to check out the possibility that it has a physical cause. If this can be eliminated, then you can proceed with a self-help program such as the one in these chapters.

If you answered *yes* to question 1, but *no* to question 2, you also should have a physical examination, again to rule out the possibility of physical cause. Even if you have had a regular physical checkup recently, you should still seek a medical opinion if you have not specifically discussed your sexual difficulties with a physician. If you are receiving medication for some condition (for example, hypertension), discuss with your doctor the possibility that your problem may be a side effect of the drug and, if so, what options are available. If your doctor feels that there is no physical basis for your sexual dysfunction, you may then pursue the program in this book with greater peace of mind.

If you answered questions 2, 4, and 5 with *yes,* the chances are small that your sexual difficulties have a physical cause, simply because you *are* able to get erections, at least under certain circumstances. You might still want to go for a physical exam, however, just to be on the safe side.

If you replied *yes* to question 2, but *no* to question 3, you need to do two things *before* you begin this program. First, you owe it to yourself to learn more about your own sexuality (see chapters 1, 2, and 4). Second, the fact that you can get erections alone, but have never had an erection during a sexual encounter, suggests that some discomfort on your part, either with women in general or their bodies in particular, may be contributing to your difficulties. To begin dealing with this issue, work through the exercises in chapter 7. Then return to this chapter and pick it up where you left off.

If you *are* able to experience erections regularly by some means of stimulation (question 2), *have* had an erection during at least one sexual encounter in the past (question 3), but *presently do not* experience erections at all in such recent situations (questions 6 and 7), then there are essentially two explanations: you are not sexually attracted to your partner, or you are attracted but something is interfering with your sexual response during your encounters with her. In the first instance, your lack of erections may simply reflect your lack of desire. This possibility is essentially confirmed if you answered *yes* to question 9. In that case, you need to start dealing with the problem by exploring this issue of sexual desire, toward an end of discovering the possible reasons for your lack of interest and also to see if some things can be changed to increase it. Chapters 1, 2, 3, and 4 have this as their goal. The other possibility, that something interferes with your sexual response when you make love, is most likely due to anxiety (nervous tension) or something related, for instance, guilt. In that case, you should stay with this program. Although it is not essential that you go back to earlier chapters as a way to start dealing with the sexual problem, you may still be referred to other parts of the book from time to time to learn specific techniques. Also, you may benefit in other ways from the material in earlier chapters, above and beyond what you get out of this one, and may want to go through them when you have time.

If your situation is that you can at least occasionally experience an erection, even temporarily, during a sexual encounter (question 6), your problem is less severe than that of a man who never experiences an erection when he is making love. Similarly, if you sometimes experience an erection that is strong enough to allow you at least to start intercourse on occasion (question 7), your situation is that much more hopeful. If this is your situation, depending on your expectations for yourself, you may not have a sexual dysfunction at all.

> Mr. X called to ask if there was a therapy program that could help him to "overcome" what he referred to as his "erection dysfunction." I suggested that he come to see me in order to assess the problem in more detail. In the course of his later interview, it was soon apparent that Mr. X and I had quite different perspectives on the "problem." His goals for therapy were two: to be able to get a second erection more quickly after an orgasm (he currently needed a pause of about an hour or so) and to be able to ejaculate with more force.
>
> Mr. X was past sixty-five years old, and although I sympathized with his desires, I felt that his concerns about his sexual performance were based on a lack of knowledge and that his goals were, as a result, unrealistic. He was in excellent health and condition for his age, but Mr. X was, in my opinion, experiencing some normal effects of aging on his sexual response. These effects include the very things he thought were a dysfunction. Specifically, as men age it takes longer for them to be able to get another erection after having an orgasm. Also, it is commonly reported that the force of ejaculation decreases gradually with age and that some older men tend to lose the sensations associated with ejaculation.

There is no good reason why anyone should have to give up his or her sex life with aging or why people should cease to enjoy sexual activity, be it alone or with a partner. It is another unfortunate myth of our culture that older people are asexual (having no sexual interests). Fortunately, progress is being made in challenging this sort of thinking, just as it is in challenging traditional views of male and female sexuality. However, the effects of age on sexuality are real, and to deny them (or be ignorant of them) can create unrealistic expectations, which set the stage, in time, for feelings of frustration and disappointment.

It should be clear from Exercise 8.1 that there are many different kinds of erection problems. The purpose of this exercise is to help you get a clearer understanding of your particular situation in relation to other men and to ascertain if you should begin trying to overcome the problem. If the suggestion that you go to some other chapter as a first step applies to you, do so as soon as you finish reading this. When you have finished that necessary groundwork, you may be in a better position to benefit from what follows in the next sections. Otherwise proceed with the exercises that follow.

EXPECTING THE POSSIBLE: SEXUAL DESIRE AND ERECTION PROBLEMS

Men sometimes do expect the impossible, or nearly that, in that they think they should be able to get an erection even when making love to someone they are not sexually attracted to. Sometimes it seems humorous, but mostly sad, to hear a man complaining about his difficulties in getting it up with a woman he obviously is not turned on to, and then concluding that there is something wrong with him because he can't. As we discussed in chapter 1, sexual myths stand in the way of sexual fulfillment and contribute to sexual dysfunctions. Some of our traditional ideas about male sexuality are particularly harmful, especially the myth that claims men are sexually insensitive and driven.

A more humane and less limiting view of human sexuality is that sexual desire, in both men and women, is more complex than simple, more delicate than rugged. Feeling sexual desire at any given time is an experience that results from an *interaction* of factors, some of which may lie inside of us and others having to do with the *situation* we are in at the time. In short, the *particular* woman, *particular* time, and *particular* place must be right for the man in order for him to feel sexual desire for that woman.

You cannot expect to get an erection if you are not feeling sexually aroused, and you cannot get sexually aroused with someone you are not attracted to. Sexual attraction, or desire, is a response in you that depends on at least two things: a feeling on your part that sex is something enjoyable and the availability of someone (either real or imagined) who fits your ideas of what is sexually appealing. When these two minimum conditions exist (that is, when a person enjoys and values sex, and sees or imagines a sexually desirable partner), he or she can experience sexual desire. When one or the other of these minimum conditions is lacking (for example, if the person does not enjoy or value sex or there are no appealing partners available), sexual interest will not happen; therefore, there is little or no chance of becoming sexually aroused. If you doubt this, talk with someone who has deliberately chosen to lead a celibate life-style. Chances are you will not find this person "starving" for sex. Similarly, you may recall periods in your own life when you were not particularly interested in sex, that is, when you didn't find it particularly enjoyable. The reason that celibates can do without sex is not that they are missing an instinct, but that they have chosen not to value sex so highly (or they have chosen to value other things more highly than sexual pleasure). By the same token, during those periods when you have been "off" sexually, the more likely explanation is not that some instinct was misplaced, but that other things were more important to you then.

The above conditions for sexual arousal were purposely described as "minimal." The reason is that having them filled is *necessary,* but it is not always *sufficient* to produce sexual arousal. Even when you do like and value sexual pleasure and have an appealing partner available, so that you do experience sexual desire, other factors may still interfere with arousal. These factors, such as anxiety, will be discussed later. For now it is more important to concentrate on the basic idea that men do not have an automatic, instinctive, and constant sex drive that is not influenced by circumstances. You as a man are not, in short, a sexual machine. Your sex drive, or desire, is the result of a complex combination of factors. Certain minimum conditions must be met for you to experience sexual desire, and potential interferences must be eliminated for you to experience arousal in a particular situation. These conditions may be easy to meet, and you may not suffer from any interfering complications, in which case your sexuality may not seem like a very sensitive or discriminating sort of thing. But this would only reflect the facts that your conditions are being met and that there are no complications. Don't be misled by this. When and if your situation changes, so that it is not so easy to meet your conditions, or if something like anxiety begins to interfere, you will, for better or worse, be in a position to appreciate your sexual sensitivities.

One basic cause of erection problems in men, then, has to do with expecting the impossible—believing that you are not sexually sensitive and expecting yourself to get turned on and perform well in situations that are not conducive to you. If you have any question as to whether you may be trying to "force" your sexual arousal, you should reread chapter 2 now before proceeding further with this program. If you honestly feel that sexual desire is not related to your difficulties, you may go on with the program. You might, however, want to look through chapter 2 at some time in the future.

COMPLICATIONS

It is true that *if* conditions are right and *if* there are no complications, a man who feels turned on to his partner will get sexually aroused and experience an erection as part of that arousal. It does not follow, however, that not having an erection means that a man is not feeling sexual desire for his partner. The fact that he is not experiencing an erection may be a sign that there is some *complication,* something that is interfering with his ability to experience an erection, even though he is feeling turned on. The next section discusses some of the possible complicating factors that can get between arousal and erection, so as to cause a sexual dysfunction.

Complication 1: Fear

Fear is an expectation of something bad happening during a sexual encounter with a particular woman. You believe that there may be some negative consequences as a result of going to bed with her. Your fear of these consequences works in opposition to your sexual arousal. Obviously, the fear can be intense or mild.

The intensity of the fear you will experience depends on two things: what the particular consequences are and how likely you think it is that they will occur. As an example, let's take pregnancy as a possible consequence of having sex. Assuming that you don't want to conceive a child at the time, it would be fair to say that your partner getting pregnant would be a highly undesirable consequence of a sexual encounter. Whether your fear will be intense or mild, however, will depend not only on how bad this prospect seems to you, but also on how likely you think it is that your partner will get pregnant. If you, she, or both use some form of birth control, and if you have confidence in its effectiveness, then your fear will naturally be less intense than if you do not use a contraceptive. For most people, then, the use of some proven means of birth control brings this particular fear down to a minimum. However, fear of pregnancy can, in some cases, be very intense so long as there is the slightest chance of it happening.

> Mr. A had been experiencing erection difficulties on and off for several years, and regularly for the previous year and a half. Earlier, his problem was that he would lose his erections as soon as intercourse started, but now he did not experience erections at all. I was convinced that he was attracted to his wife, but she had come to doubt her appeal and was feeling down about herself at this point.
>
> Mr. A, an executive, and his wife had six children in the fifteen years of their marriage. Both the second and the last time she got pregnant, Mrs. A had been using a diaphragm regularly. Mr. A found the responsibilities of his family and household to be a considerable burden, which was made even heavier by his own desire to live almost grandly. As you might guess, this, in addition to his job, made for a high pressure existence. At the time of our meeting, the last thing the A's wanted was to have another child. Also, although Mrs. A may have gotten pregnant those two times because she was prescribed a diaphragm that did not fit her well or because she used it incorrectly, correcting these possibilities (through a new fitting) did not lead to any improvement in Mr. A's functioning, nor did my suggestion that they each use some form of birth control (a condom for him, plus her diaphragm). Suggesting that they agree not to have intercourse, but to go to bed and engage in a sensual massage (as described in chapter 6) did result in Mr. A getting erections. But as soon as I suggested that they try letting Mrs. A get on top and insert her husband's penis into her vagina, his erections, even during the massages, disappeared. It soon became clear that the reason for this setback was his fear of pregnancy. Because of his past experiences, my approach was not successful in reducing this fear, that is, of convincing Mr. A that it was now safe to have sex with his wife. Not only would having another child be an extremely undesirable consequence for him, but he held a belief that his wife was so fertile that no amount of birth control would be enough.
>
> We discussed the difficulty and the setback, and I shared my impressions of the causes of difficulty with the couple. Over a

period of weeks and after considering all the options together, Mr. A opted to undergo a vasectomy. Although Mrs. A had considered a tubal ligation (having her "tubes tied"), Mr. A actually felt he would feel safest if he took the necessary step rather than his wife.

After he recovered from the surgery, we picked up the sex therapy where we had left off, and Mr. A was soon experiencing erections again during sensual massages. This time when I suggested that Mrs. A get on top and insert her husband's penis, he did not lose his erection. Apparently, he was finally convinced that he no longer had to fear sex, and so his natural sexual response took over.

Fear is based on an apprehension of some *real* and *undesirable* consequence. Pregnancy, for example, is real, and it can be highly undesirable. Other real and undesirable consequences of sex may concern embarrassment; some people, for instance, fear getting caught "in the act" by a jealous spouse or their own children. So long as they expect that this is likely to happen and feel that it would be a terrible thing if it did happen, such men are likely to suffer sexual consequences when they try to have a sexual encounter, even if they have a lot of sexual desire for their partners.

Yet another form of fear has to do with the *implications* of sex for your relationship with a particular woman.

Mr. B was a bachelor in his early forties. He described himself as a man who had had many girlfriends, but few serious relationships. Twice for brief periods he had lived with women, but as he initially described them, these "experiments" didn't work out.

Mr. B's sexual problem concerned his longstanding difficulties in getting and maintaining erections. Moreover, at the time he came to see me, he had not had a date in more than two years. He attributed this to his fear of "failing" sexually and to the embarrassment this would cause him. Although this seemed true enough, it later seemed that Mr. B had yet a second fear, which had to do with involvement. He had always been a shy, unassertive person. At the same time, he was attractive and fairly well off financially. He had few friends, and by-and-large preferred to spend his free time in pursuit of solitary hobbies, such as reading, carpentry, and gardening.

Although it was true that he had had many girlfriends, he never really felt comfortable around women. In fact, he had always perceived them as more powerful then he in that he found it difficult to stand up for himself and was hesitant to do or say anything that might cause hurt feelings. As a result he often felt that he was getting in over his head in relationships. For example, on the two occasions when he supposedly "experimented" with sharing his house, it turned out to be more the woman's idea than his. Of course, he was not completely innocent in these doings. For one thing, he never gave either woman the slightest hint that he did not want to live with her. At the same time, he probably did at least hint that he might like it. Nevertheless, I was inclined to believe that this was so largely because he was so unassertive and, therefore, felt so helpless around women.

As part of this helplessness, Mr. B also tended to feel anxious about having a sexual relationship with a woman. He feared that this would imply some commitment to her on his part. Whenever he went to bed with a woman, he would think about whether she would take it to mean he loved her and wanted to share his life with her. I was certain that this sort of worrying was a major contribution to his erection problem. After a while he began to feel this way, too, and realized that he needed to work on becoming more assertive in general, and with women in particular. By learning that he had a right to set some limits, for himself at least, on a relationship and by working toward being more up-front and open about his desires, he could work his way out of fearing sex because of what it could get him into.

A sexual encounter between two people is seldom a purely physical experience. Having a sexual encounter may imply nothing more about your relationship with a woman other than that you like each others' bodies, but it rarely means only this.

For many people—perhaps the majority—it means much more. It can, in some cases, be taken to mean that you are making a firm commitment to the relationship. An expectation on your part, that by going to bed with someone you may be getting in over your head in terms of commitment, is a fear that quite a number of men seem to have. At times this particular fear can be so great that it will interfere with your ability to get sexually aroused even when you are feeling very turned on to your partner.

To overcome a fear that is interfering with your ability to experience erections during sexual encounters, you need to consider both components of the fear, as mentioned earlier. First, you need to assess just how bad the consequence really is. Second, you need to look at how likely it is that the consequence will occur. You may then need to take action in one or both of these areas. If making your sexual partner pregnant is something that is very undesirable to you, you need to minimize the chances of that happening or to agree between you and your partner on what you will do if it does happen. If you fear being found out, you can try to insure your privacy, reconsider just how bad that sort of thing would be, or both, and so on. In short, if the consequence really would be terrible from your point of view, you can only reduce your fear by minimizing the chances of it happening. In most cases, this is possible to do if you (and your partner) are willing to take responsibility for doing it. Considering all of the alternatives available today, the possibilities of pregnancy, for example, can be virtually eliminated if sufficient care is taken by the two of you.

Sometimes it may be impossible to eliminate a possibility completely. For example, there is no way that you can be certain, in advance, that a woman won't become more emotionally involved with you than you are with her as a result of having a sexual relationship. Even if you make it clear ahead of time that having sex does not, for you, necessarily mean you're in love, a woman may still feel strongly about you after your relationship has become more intimate, and she will be disappointed at best if her feelings are not returned. In this case, you need to consider the issue of responsibility, as well as just how bad such a thing would be. Are someone else's feelings about you totally your doing or do people have to take some responsibility for their own feelings? Is it really a terrible thing (that *you* have done) if someone becomes more involved with you than you are with them, and ends up hurt or disappointed? People are responsible, at most, for being honest with one another, and people's feelings for each other can change, often very quickly. Therefore, there is no way to be sure ahead of time that someone will feel the way you want them to about you.

If fear is your problem, remember that it amounts to an expectation that something bad is going to happen. The feared consequence is real. The intensity of the fear (and the likelihood that it will interfere with your sexual performance) depends largely on how bad the consequence is in your own mind and how likely you think it is to happen if you have sex. Naturally, the worse the consequence and the more likely you think it is, the worse your fear will be. Dealing with your fear, then, may involve an attempt to reduce one or both of the factors that contribute to it. Usually people try to minimize the chances of the consequence occurring, but it is also possible to reevaluate consequences to see if they really are as bad as you think.

Complication 2: Guilt
Guilt is a feeling that what you are doing is wrong or sinful. It can, like fear, interfere with your sexual response, causing an erection problem even when you are feeling a lot of sexual desire. Like fear, guilt usually exerts its effects after you have experienced sexual desire, that is, after you already feel turned on. It then works to undermine your level of arousal. The result is that you feel sexually excited but, if the guilt is strong enough, you do not experience an erection.

Between guilt and fear, guilt seems the more difficult complication to deal with. Although it may be popular today, at least in some circles, to say that guilt is a bad thing—something to be gotten rid of, period—that is much too simple a way to look at it. Our sense of morality (of what is "right" and what is "wrong") is a very important part of being human, and it would be a mistake to throw it out the window, even if we could. What seems more reasonable is that, as adults, each of us needs to reassess the morality we more or less swallowed whole as children. This is anything but simple to do, and reevaluating values with respect to sex may be the most difficult of all.

The central idea you need to embrace is that physical, sexual pleasure is something that every person has a right to. If you detect a shade of doubt in yourself in regard to this belief, or if that statement makes you hesitate, one reason may be that you have some guilty feelings about sex. If your response to the idea that we all have a right to sexual pleasure is wholehearted agreement, then turn your attention to considering your ideas about what *kinds* of sexual pleasure are right and which, if any, are wrong. For example, is it all right to give sexual pleasure to yourself, or is it only okay if someone else gives it to you? Men generally have somewhat permissive attitudes toward self-pleasure, but some do feel it is wrong. As one older man put it, "Nature didn't intend that thing to be a plaything." This particular man's sex guilt was so strong that he could not touch himself even to see if he could give himself an erection (as a way of eliminating the chances that the problem had a physical cause); nor could he say the word *penis* even after I used it several times and we were alone.

Feeling uncomfortable about sex is not an easy complication to overcome. There are, however, several things you can try. First, read or reread chapters 2 and 4 and do the exercises in them. If you are a religious person, you might find it helpful to discuss your feelings about sex with at least two priests, ministers, or rabbis. Today there are few members of the clergy who would be truly surprised, much less angry or disapproving, that you have some concerns in this area. There are also a number of books on sex written by and for religious people. These should be available in many religious and other bookstores.

Following is one particular type of guilt that I have encountered several times.

> Mr. C was a man in his early forties. He had been married for seventeen years, but he was, at the time I saw him, separated from his wife. The separation had been in effect for only a few months, but already Mr. C was deeply involved with another woman. Although he felt he loved this woman very much, Mr. C had never been able to experience an erection with her. He had occasionally had erection difficulties during his marriage, usually at times when he and his wife were not getting along, but he had never experienced the sort of difficulty he was having now. After talking with me for a while, Mr. C found himself wondering out loud if his problem might not be due to guilt. As he put it, somehow it just didn't feel right to him to be having sex with someone he wasn't married to. Later it came out that he also felt guilty about having left his wife and children and saw himself as a bad person for having done so.

Here is a similar case.

> Mr. D, in his fifties, had lost his wife to a prolonged illness almost a year before coming to see me. Since his wife's death, he had tried to have sexual relations with several women, but he was never able to get an erection during these encounters. He was both upset and puzzled, since before his wife's death he had had an affair that he found sexually fulfilling and in which he never experienced erection difficulties. This affair broke up just a few months before he lost his wife, when his lover decided to move to another part of the country.
>
> After talking with Mr. D for a while, it occurred to me that he was not especially depressed, but that he did feel very uncomfortable about his affair, as well as a couple of others he had had during the course of his marriage. He felt, I guessed, guilty about

having cheated on a sick woman and he probably would not have seen it from my prospective, which was that the extramarital relationship provided him with needed pleasure as well as support and relief from the burdens of caretaking.

When I suggested my "interpretation" to Mr. D, he reacted with a lot of emotion. It was a moving experience for both of us.

The sort of guilt that Mr. C and Mr. D were experiencing seems to respond best to two things, the first of which is time. The adage that "time heals" seems true, and if you feel that your situation is similar to either of the above men, first of all, give yourself some time. Continue to pursue relationships with women you want to be with. Accept the facts that it will take some time for your wounds to heal and that as your bad feelings fade, your sexual performance may recover.

The second thing that might be helpful to men in these positions is to keep in mind that you have not only responsibilities to others in life, but also a responsibility to yourself. Neither Mr. C or Mr. D seemed to feel that they had a right to some happiness of their own. We raise men and women alike to have a strong sense of responsibility to others, their spouses, children, and families. Although there is value in the concept of social responsibility, there are limits to the responsibilities we have to others; at some point we need to take care of ourselves, too.

Guilt, in sum, is a complication whereby you feel that what you are doing is wrong or sinful. The roots lie in our upbringings, where we develop a sense of morality that we later use to judge our own behavior. Although they are important, our personal values can also lead us to judge ourselves too harshly. This seems especially true in the area of sex, where our traditional attitudes have led many of us to grow up feeling that sex is somehow dirty, sinful, or shameful.

Guilt that interferes with a person's sexual response usually reflects his or her feeling that sex is wrong *under particular circumstances*. Obviously, there are then only two possible ways to deal with it: you can reassess your attitudes and decide that your behavior is not wrong, or you can try to change the circumstances. Usually, people try to change the circumstances rather than trying to rethink their attitudes, since morals tend to be deeply ingrained and not easily altered. However difficult it may be, there may be much to gain from such a personal reassessment.

Complication 3: Resentment and Jealousy

A third complication that can enter the picture and interfere with your sexual arousal is a feeling of resentment and/or jealousy.

> Mr. E, in his late thirties, had been divorced for nearly five years. During the few months immediately following his initial separation from his wife, he experienced sexual difficulties, mainly premature ejaculation. Over time these difficulties subsided and for the next few years the only problems he had concerned losing his erections or getting only partial erections, usually during the first few encounters he had with a new sexual partner. This is nothing unusual for men and would not be considered a sexual dysfunction. Since he preferred to date only one or two women at a time and to maintain relationships for a while, this tendency for "opening night jitters" as he put it, did not bother Mr. E a great deal, although he certainly wished it could be different.
>
> The reason Mr. E came to see me had nothing to do with this pattern, but rather with the fact that, suddenly, and for the past several months, he had been experiencing a lot of difficulty getting and keeping erections. His overall situation at that time was that he had become seriously involved with a woman he had been seeing for about a year, to the point that they were now considering living together. He felt certain that this was what he wanted to do and was looking forward to it.
>
> Sexually, however, his erection problems were getting worse. He thought he knew what was responsible for it but he was afraid to discuss his feelings with his partner. It seemed that

when they were in bed together, he found himself thinking about his partner's former lovers. He would compare himself to what he imagined they were like or he would imagine his partner making love to one of them, and then he would lose his erection. All of these interfering thoughts had started around the same time that the relationship moved to a more serious level. Before then, he never felt put off by thoughts of his partner's previous lovers; in fact, since his divorce he had found discussions of past affairs, by both himself and his lovers, to be interesting and even a turn-on. Now, however, he was not finding sex talk at all enjoyable, at least not when the topic was previous men his partner had been involved with. He felt that what he was doing was silly—that he did not have any reason to fear or be jealous of his partner's ex-lovers, or to be angry at her—but he felt helpless at the same time to do anything about it.

Men in our culture are raised to be very competitive. One of the prime things we compete over is women. As the saying goes, we try to "win" a partner, and once we do that, she becomes personal property in our minds. Besides physical beauty, one of the things that has always been prized in a woman is her sexual history; the less sexual experience she has had, the more a woman has traditionally been valued, with attractive virgins being valued most highly of all. The man who competed with other men for a beautiful virgin and "won" her has, therefore, been respected and admired by other men. Men take women to be such strong symbols of their own worth that for a long time it was not considered a crime for a man to kill his wife if he caught her in the act with another man, and dying women who confessed to an affair had their gravestones later marked to set them apart from their more virtuous peers.

Our culture is in the process of challenging some of its traditional values, and the idea that women are valuable property that men should compete over and then own is one of these values. Women, by and large, no longer wish to belong to a man in the same way a car or a horse can belong to him. The change in values is far from complete, however, and as Mr. E's dilemma illustrates men (and women) still have a long way to go.

For Mr. E, I saw two ways to deal with the problem. On the one hand, he could reassess things and decide that his partner really was not a piece of property that could be owned, now that they were serious, any more than she was when they were simply dating. If he could accept the fact that he did not own her, then the fact that she had lovers before him could not be taken as a reflection on his or her worth. Getting involved with this woman was not, in short, like buying a car, in which case getting something brand new reflects better on you than getting something secondhand.

The other alternative available to Mr. E is time. Simply put, he might be able to forget about his partner's former lovers after a while without ever changing his basic attitudes. That is, he can go on thinking of his partner as his property, but he may come to forget the fact that she had "previous owners." Whichever alternative he chose—changing his attitudes or letting time pass—as his interfering jealousy dissipated, Mr. E's erection problem would probably also improve.

As the following example shows, resentment can operate in a way similar to jealousy to sabotage a man's sexual arousal.

> Mr. F was in his late twenties, married, and the father of two young children. He was devoted to his family, felt very much in love with his wife, and was committed to his career. About a year before he saw me, Mr. F's father-in-law died. Six months after the death, his mother-in-law moved in. As we talked I realized, mainly from little things he said rather than from pointed complaints, that Mr. F had agreed to this mainly to please his wife, and out of a general sense of responsibility. Personally, he had always found his wife's mother a bit obnoxious and living with her had not done anything to change his opinion. The mother-daughter relationship, meanwhile, was close, and he understandably felt like an outsider. Worse, if a conflict did break out, he felt that his wife would take her mother's side over

his. So far there had been no major conflicts but many little ones, and Mr. F believed he was getting the short end of the stick. At first, this was only slightly annoying and his anger would quickly subside. After a while, however, his inner reactions became stronger, and he became more and more hesitant to express his feelings to his wife or mother-in-law.

When he first started to experience problems getting and keeping erections during their sexual encounters, neither Mr. F nor his wife worried a lot about it. They had never had a very active sex life together, and he had occasionally had such difficulties before, usually when the pressures of work got high. These occasional difficulties, however, never lasted longer than one or two sexual encounters. Now the situation was much different—Mr. F had not been able to maintain an erection long enough to complete intercourse for about three months—and they were both worried. Meanwhile, in the months since Mrs. F's mother had been with them, the marriage had become cool. When I saw them, they seemed uncomfortable with each other, which was not at all the way Mr. F had described his marriage, and he acted much differently—stiff and tense—than he had when I initially spoke with him alone.

Oddly enough, neither Mr. F nor his wife had personally made any connection between the events of the previous year and his sexual difficulties. To say that he had a sexual dysfunction, which was how they saw the problem, was simply missing the boat. What he *and* his wife had, as a couple, was a marital crisis, precipitated by the addition of the mother-in-law to the household. I believed that the feelings of resentment Mr. F felt in response to his position within the family, especially when it came to conflicts, were the basis for his erection difficulties. Therefore, the solution to the problem was to be found, first of all, in resolving the marital crisis that he (and his wife) was avoiding. Then if the erection difficulties continued, say, because of performance anxiety (discussed later), we could deal with it directly, using the desensitization procedure described in chapter 9. Probably because his sexual attitudes toward himself were good and because his wife did love him and wanted to help, his difficulties did disappear once the main marital conflict was resolved.

Jealousy and resentment are two additional feelings that can complicate a man's sexual response, undermining his performance even when he feels turned on. Resentment, when it is present and interfering with things, is a sign that there is an open (or hidden) conflict between you and your partner. Generally, unspoken or hidden conflicts are more damaging to a sexual relationship than are conflicts that are out in the open. In dealing with resentments, therefore, a first goal would be to express them so that you and your partner know what you are dealing with. The next step, of course, is to attempt to resolve the conflict—to try to come up with some sort of solution. Sometimes just being able to complain or get angry is enough of a resolution. At other times you will need to reach some sort of compromise solution. In the case of Mr. and Mrs. F, the solution to his discomfort in the end was to arrange for his mother-in-law to take a small apartment of her own, with their financial assistance, in the same neighborhood. That way she could be close to her daughter and grandchildren, but not so close as to disrupt the marriage.

There are a few ways to deal with jealousy. For one, if there is something your partner is doing that arouses your jealousy, she may be willing to stop it. If she enjoys flirting with other men, for instance, and if this gets you upset, she may be willing to stop that in the interests of your relationship. Like resentment, jealousy needs to be expressed—to be out in the open—before it can be dealt with. Jealousy that seems based largely in your partner's past experiences cannot be relieved by anything she can do in the present, except perhaps to reassure you that she loves you. In this instance, the solution lies within yourself, if there is to be one. Two courses are open—you can wait for time to cool you down or you can reassess the attitudes that are the basis for your jealousy. In either case, the solution to the problem of jealousy is often an essential element in the treatment of sexual difficulties.

Complication 4: Sexual Phobias

Your sexual response, and specifically your ability to experience an erection, can also be sabotaged by a sexual phobia, which can vary from mild feelings of discomfort with women's bodies, on the one hand, to intense reactions like disgust on the other. Often a sexual phobia does not prevent a man from feeling sexually attracted to a woman; that is, he can still experience sexual desire. It does, however, interfere with his sexual arousal once he is in an actual sexual encounter. Usually his reaction of uneasiness is specific to the woman's naked body, and often even more specifically to her breasts and/or genitals.

> Mr. G was a single man in his early twenties. He came to see me, feeling very upset, because of what had happened two days earlier. He had a sexual encounter and, as usual, did not get an erection.
>
> Mr. G and his lover had been seeing one another regularly for about six months, and even though they had gone to bed often, he never got an erection. Privately he was aware that he did not enjoy looking at, or touching, his partner's genitals, and that this had been true for all the women he had been with. That his reaction to the female genitals was one of discomfort was apparent from the expression on his face when he talked about it.
>
> Since he avoided touching her, never tried oral sex, and was no doubt awkward and stiff when it came to foreplay, Mr. G's girlfriend had suspected the truth from the very beginning although he continued to deny it whenever she asked. Eventually she became so frustrated, not only because of his phobia but also because of his evasiveness and denial, that she let out her anger on that night two days earlier by accusing him of being gay. Since Mr. G himself suspected (and feared) that his aversion

to women's genitals meant that he might be homosexual, the accusation sent him into a panic.

In talking with Mr. G, I felt there was no question that he was sexually attracted to his lover, at least when she was clothed. He had already had several close, loving relationships with women, and if anything was prone to becoming very involved too quickly. Raised by very religious, rigid parents he had developed a nervous attitude toward sex at an early age. In addition, he did not feel that comfortable with his own body and tended to dress and groom rather modestly. By his own account he could not understand why he was so intensely attracted to women when they had their clothes on, but not when he went to bed with them, and he believed that there was something seriously wrong with him.

Mr. G had a genital phobia, a feeling of discomfort about the female body. These reactions often can interfere with erections, but not always with sexual desire. If you feel that part of your own problem may be due to such discomfort, the exercises in chapter 7 can be helpful to you. Do them now before going further with this program.

Complication 5: Distraction

Chapter 6 deals with the problem, which many people complain of, of not being able to relax during sexual encounters. One reason for this difficulty has to do with being distracted during lovemaking. By having something other than what is going on between you and your partner on your mind at the same time that you are making love, your level of sexual arousal decreases. One consequence of this can be a loss or a total absence of an erection. Again this may not be due to any lack of desire on your part, but due to a decreased sexual arousal because of straying thoughts.

Having your sexual arousal and performance undermined by various distractions seems a particularly common occurrence.

Mr. H was an investment counselor whose job was both lucrative and very demanding. When I met with him and his wife about his erection problem, the national economy happened to be receding. Mr. H's livelihood and the welfare of his family depended on his ability to manage the accounts of his clients successfully. With the economy in a slump and such high stakes in the balance, the pressures on Mr. H were considerable. At home, where he normally rested and escaped from these pressures, his wife found him becoming more and more irritable in general, and with her in particular. Fortunately, she was sympathetic and supportive, and they managed to work through his concerns by talking about them often. However, Mr. H then began to experience difficulties keeping his erection, and about half of the time he didn't get one at all.

During our in-depth discussion of their sexual relationship, Mrs. H commented at one point that she thought her husband's behavior in bed had changed. She thought he was still attracted to her (although she recently had begun having doubts), but that he wasn't, in her words, involved with what was going on. She thought that it might be because of his erection problem, but Mr. H said that it wasn't. He said that he had found himself worrying, in bed with his wife as much as anywhere, about his job. In fact, anytime it seemed that he started to relax, he would soon find that his mind had wandered to his accounts. Rather than relaxing or making love, he would give in to this urge, go over the day's business, and plan for the next.

Mrs. H was surprised. She hadn't any idea of what had been happening. Mr. H was embarrassed. He didn't like admitting to being so preoccupied with work. What is more, it hadn't occurred to him that this tendency might have something to do with his erection difficulties.

Mr. H's case illustrates how distractions work to sabotage a sexual experience, even when you approach it feeling very turned on. If you think about it, this makes a lot of sense. It is just about impossible to concentrate on two things at the same time. To get sexually aroused and to maintain that arousal, you must be able to focus your attention on things that are sexually *exciting*, for example, your partner's body, her responses to you, and your own body sensations when she touches you. You can also focus on sexually exciting *thoughts*, for instance, a sexual fantasy or imagining you and your partner making love. However, if you set your attention on something that is not sexually exciting, like work or the next day's shopping, you can expect your level of arousal to drop. The situation is, of course, even worse if you focus your attention on things that arouse negative feelings—for instance, if you worry—as Mr. H did.

> Mr. J was about to marry for the second time. He originally had come to therapy for help with an erection problem that seemed to be linked mainly to jealousy and guilt. The guilt came from feelings about breaking up his first marriage and the jealousy had to do with other men his future wife had dated before she met him. As a consequence of his difficulties, Mr. J developed a good deal of sexual performance anxiety, a fear of having sexual difficulties, which, in turn, only makes sexual difficulties more likely.
>
> In dealing with Mr. J's problem, we needed to address all the factors, or complications—the guilt, the jealousy, and the performance anxiety. This took a while, but it seemed to be working out when Mr. J suddenly had a setback; it happened as soon as he left his apartment and moved into his future wife's home. This time he diagnosed the complication for himself, although he didn't know what to do about it. He was intensely attracted to his fiancé and was sure that he wanted to marry her, so he had eliminated for himself the possibility that the problem was due to a lack of desire or attraction. He also felt that he had come a long way toward overcoming his guilt and jealousy and that they were no longer undermining his arousal. The problem, rather, was his fiancé's twelve-year-old son.
>
> Mr. J had never had sex in his fiancé's house when her son was there. Usually they would make love in his apartment, or in her house when they were alone. Although this seemed to reflect a shared fear (about being overheard or caught in the act), both

partners apparently chose to ignore this. Of course, as soon as Mr. J moved in, it was no longer possible to do so. He did anything but ignore it. He found himself preoccupied with thoughts of the boy: Where was he? Could he hear them? Could he see them? Understandably, his sexual arousal was sabotaged very effectively, with the result that he had trouble once more getting an erection.

Although both Mr. H's and Mr. J's problems could rightly be said to result from fear perhaps even more than simple distraction, they are included here to illustrate the general idea that having other things on your mind, worries or not, will take away from your enjoyment of a sexual encounter and reduce your level of arousal. You cannot pay attention to two things at the same time—what your lover is doing to you and whether you left your keys in the car. As a consequence of not focusing on something sexually exciting, your arousal will decline. You may not be able to get aroused enough to experience an erection, or you may lose it when your mind begins to wander.

Strategies for dealing with a tendency to be distracted during sex are described in detail in chapter 6. Briefly, you need to work on doing three things. You must try to establish a pattern of tending to business and other issues *before* making love. You must eliminate sources of distraction whenever possible—put a lock on the door! And you must develop a habit of catching yourself when you are becoming distracted and redirecting your attention to something that contributes to, rather than takes away from, your sexual arousal. Focus your attention on your body sensations as your partner touches you, on your partner's body and her responses to you, or on a sexually exciting thought.

Complication 6: Performance Anxiety

Although it is discussed last, performance anxiety is probably the most common of all complications that can interfere with sex. This is not the first time we have mentioned performance anxiety, but it is important enough to be worth reviewing.

Mr. K was in his early fifties and married to his second wife for more than fifteen years. For about three years before they sought therapy, the K's sexual relationship had steadily withered to the point where they had attempted intercourse only once in the previous year and a half. This was because of Mr. K's difficulties in keeping an erection. He would sometimes get a partial erection during foreplay. At that point he would immediately try to insert his partially erect penis into his wife's vagina, only to find that he would promptly lose the erection. The problem dated back to the time when Mr. K was diagnosed by his physician as having high blood pressure. He was prescribed a medication known to be associated with erection problems (that is, erection problems were one of its possible side effects) in some men, and in his case this apparently happened. Mr. K began having problems with his erections right after he started taking the drug. He complained to his physician (but not until nearly a year had gone by), who modified the dosage but did not change to a different medication.

Mr. K's problem continued. The situation in bed was so humiliating to him that he gradually avoided sex rather than going through the frustration and embarrassment. His wife did not want to be the one to put him through such an ordeal so she, too, avoided suggesting or otherwise initiating any sexual contact. Between the two of them, they eventually got to a point where sex just dropped out of their relationship. This, in turn, had effects on both of them and their marriage. Mr. K became irritable, overweight, and moody; Mrs. K also let herself go physically and came to feel negatively about herself as a woman.

Six months before coming to therapy, Mr. K finally changed doctors and was given a new medication for high blood pressure. He then approached his wife for sex for the first time in a year. Again he got a partial erection during foreplay. His performance anxiety, which was low going into the encounter (because of his faith in the safety of the new medication), rose immediately when he found himself with an erection. He worried about it lasting, and for fear that it would not, he went back to his old pattern of trying to enter his wife right away. As you might guess the erection disappeared, leading to a very upsetting scene and a lot of hurt feelings.

Initially Mr. K's erection problem probably had a physical cause—the medication for his blood pressure. One might suspect that the second drug he was given could have been responsible for the problem continuing but later events disproved this theory. Mr. K's problem, after his medication was changed, had to do with performance anxiety—worrying about his sexual performance. By worrying so much about it, he defeated himself.

Being afraid of losing your erection, which is another way of looking at performance anxiety, can sabotage your sexual arousal and cause an erection problem also. It sets up a vicious cycle; some initial problem leads to worry, which leads to more problems. The exercises in chapter 9 will help you overcome an erection problem by allowing you to proceed in a way that will minimize or eliminate performance anxiety. These exercises assume that your erection problem, although it may have had additional causes in the beginning, is mainly the result of performance anxiety now, and that you are feeling sexually attracted to your partner.

Complications that can interfere with your sexual performance, such as those described in this chapter, should be dealt with before you proceed with the program in chapter 9. Also, the following section concerns some issues you need to think about, and perhaps do something about, before attempting to treat yourself.

STUMBLING BLOCKS TO SUCCESS

Chances are that if you are reading this book today, your erection problems did not start yesterday. It is more likely that you have been having problems for a while, maybe years.

Perhaps things have gradually gotten worse or maybe they have always been the same. In either case, you have probably put off doing something about them for some time. This is not unusual. No man is eager to admit, even to himself, that he has a sexual problem, or that he can use some help in solving it. Men more than women prefer to think that they can (and ought to) handle problems by themselves, including sexual difficulties.

Once a man finally does admit to himself that he has a problem that won't go away and decides at last to take the difficult step of seeking outside help (even from a book), he usually expects too much, too soon. He thinks things should improve immediately. Although their impatience is understandable, men can and do defeat themselves this way. Rather than feeling good about slow but steady progress, they get impatient and want an immediate "cure." So, they go to a therapist, hoping that he can give them a shot or some pills that will make the problem disappear overnight. I have also been asked quite often to use hypnosis on men who think that there is some such quick, almost magical solution to their difficulties. Such men make their situation worse for themselves. The first point here is that the program in chapters 8 and 9 is less likely to work if you move through it too quickly, if you skip steps, or if you become impatient with your progress. If you are to benefit from it as much as possible, you must be willing to confront your impatience and keep it in check.

A second stumbling block to success in helping yourself has to do with the kind of relationship you have with the woman who will be your partner in this effort. For this program to be most effective, it is best if you go through it with just *one* particular sexual partner. Obviously, if you are married or living with someone, that partner should be your wife or lover. If you are living with someone, but don't feel you can (or want to) ask her to be your partner in these exercises, you ought to be asking yourself why. Is the problem that you are afraid to ask for help? Sometimes a man may feel that it would be placing a great burden on his partner to ask her to do the things described in the exercises in this book. Actually, the burden you will be placing on her is the same one you must carry yourself—the ability to cooperate and to be patient. In reality few women are actually put off by what the exercises ask them to do; more typically, they enjoy them a great deal.

Another reason why men may hesitate to ask their partners to work on these exercises with them is that they expect, and fear, a negative reaction of another sort, that their partners will find the exercises morally objectionable. If this is true, then your partner may have sexual inhibitions that contribute to your problem. If she would like to loosen up a bit, the exercises in chapters 1, 2, 3, and 4 may be as useful to her as they were to you, and you might suggest she read them. If she is unwilling to go at least that far, or if she continues to find the exercises offensive, then it may be more difficult for you to overcome your own problem. If you expect resistance from your partner, ask her to read this book and think about it before you ask her to work with you. Try to come to an agreement between you as to what sorts of sexual goals you would like to set for yourselves, as individuals and as a couple.

Yet another response from men who say they could not ask their partners to do these exercises (and especially those in chapter 9,) is that they expect their partners will find it all very one-sided, in other words, that the man will get more than the woman. This is simply not true. The program outlined does *not* neglect the woman. However, it does ask her to be as patient as you need her to be, and it also asks that she take part of the responsibility for your sexual fulfillment as a couple. The exercises involve a good deal of give-and-take, and they assume that you do want to share responsibility. In this sense they involve a departure from the active man/passive woman sexual script you may be used to. It may take both of you some time to adjust to a fifty-fifty sexual arrangement, but clearly the program is not based on selfishness nor is it one-sided.

If you do ask your wife or lover to participate as your partner in the program, your success will be largely a function of how well you can work cooperatively on each of the various steps it involves. If your relationship is strained or hostile, or if your partner is participating unwillingly, this is bound to have negative effects on how well you do. You don't need to have a perfect relationship (there are none anyway), but you do need to be able to set aside your conflicts and work together for an hour or so, a couple of times a week, if the program is to have a chance of succeeding. This would, of course, also be true if you were to go for sex therapy instead of using a book.

If you are a single man living alone, the issue of a partner is more complicated. Certainly the one thing you should *not* do is approach a woman and begin a relationship *solely* to find a partner for the program. Many women will justifiably feel offended at being asked to base a relationship on such terms. If you are close with a woman, and if sex has been a part of that relationship, you should feel free to broach the topic of going through the program together. You both stand to gain in the long run, and the exercises will be pleasurable in many ways for both of you. It would be better for both of you, however, if you could talk about what doing exercises from the book together might mean for your relationship. It doesn't necessarily have to do so, but working together on such exercises can bring you a lot closer. If you definitely do not want to risk getting closer to one another, you ought to wait until you have another partner available.

Single men who are having sexual difficulties often end up avoiding women simply because they don't want to be embarrassed by the sexual problem. In a very real sense they end up with two problems to overcome—their erection difficulty and their sexual shyness. Of these problems, avoidance of women needs to be dealt with first. (Chapter 6 can help you to do this.)

If you have been avoiding women sexually but feel ready to resume your social life, the same caution still applies with respect to approaching a woman solely with the intent of getting a partner for the exercises in this book. It would be better for you to approach a woman simply because you like her and would like to spend some time with her. You may decide to tell her about your sexual difficulties before you ever get close to having a sexual encounter, or you may decide to say nothing, have a sexual encounter, and see what happens. In either case, you would be better off developing something of a relationship before attempting to work cooperatively on your erection difficulties.

When you do feel that you know a woman whom you like well enough, and who you think might be willing to be your partner in this program (or any other in the book), ask her to read all of the material ahead of time. Give her some time to think about it and then talk together about doing it. Share your feelings, both positive and negative. If you decide to go ahead, you will be starting off on the right foot.

SUMMARY

This chapter focuses specifically on the issue of erection problems, difficulties in getting or keeping erections during sexual encounters. This is a particularly upsetting problem for a man to experience, partly because of the limitations that a nonerect penis places on a sexual encounter, but mainly because of the importance and meaning that people place on an erect penis. Erection problems often cause men to question their masculinity, women their attractiveness. Because of the importance you place on having an erection, difficulties of this sort frequently lead to performance anxiety and a vicious cycle in which worrying about your erection causes you to lose your sexual arousal and your erection.

Traditional myths about the nature of male sexuality can set the stage for erection problems by leading men to expect too much of themselves. Having an erection is not a matter of pure instinct. It is a response in you that depends on many factors and which can be interfered with by many factors. On the simplest level, to experience an erection you need to feel sexually aroused (turned on), and in order to feel sexually aroused, you need to feel sexual desire for a particular woman, at a particular time, under particular circumstances. Expecting yourself to be able to get aroused with a woman you are not interested in, or under circumstances that are not to your liking, is self-defeating.

Even when you are feeling turned on to a particular woman, it is possible for your sexual arousal, hence your erection, to be undermined by any number of factors: some consequence of sex that you fear; a feeling that what you are doing is wrong; or distraction. These factors often are responsible for erection problems *beginning,* and they therefore need to be dealt with.

Once a man has experienced erection difficulties, whatever the cause, he frequently gets himself into a position of worrying about his sexuality. This is performance anxiety, and it is what is most often responsible for an erection problem *continuing*. The problem of performance anxiety and how to deal with it is the subject of the next chapter.

9 dealing with erection problems

Since this chapter is a continuation of chapter 8, if you are a man who is experiencing problems getting or maintaining erections, be sure to read chapter 8 before this one. It includes exercises designed to help you understand your particular difficulty better and to start you on the road to overcoming it.

The program in this chapter is aimed at helping you overcome your erection problem by minimizing sexual performance anxiety—the fear a man may have that his penis won't get erect or that he will lose his erection during a sexual encounter. This fear, of course, is based on actual experience in having such difficulties, which may have been caused by things that have nothing to do with performance anxiety. However, this program is based on the assumption that this form of anxiety, which can also be thought of as self-consciousness, *becomes* a cause of erection problems. That is, we assume that worrying about your penis and what will happen to it contributes to an erection problem even after the original causes for some difficulties are no longer present. This happens because worrying self-consciously about your erection is *not* a sexually exciting thought; therefore, your level of arousal declines, and with it goes your erection. To solve the problem, you need some way to break this sort of vicious cycle in which worrying about problems brings them on.

Although it seems that performance anxiety contributes to *maintaining* erection problems, it is also true that the reasons for the *initial* difficulties a man can experience might not have anything to do with worrying about his sexual performance. These initial problems with getting or keeping erections can have any number of causes, as the following diagram suggests. These causes, discussed in chapter 8, include lack of sexual desire, as well as complicating or interfering factors, such as fear, guilt, resentment, jealousy, discomfort with women's bodies, and being distracted. Any one (or any combination) of these factors could be responsible for some initial erection difficulties. Sexual performance anxiety comes into play *later on,* after the initial difficulties have occurred. Performance anxiety, or self-conscious worry, works to turn these initial difficulties into a more or less permanent sexual dysfunction.

It is important that the causes of erection difficulties not be overlooked, since they may still be factors actively contributing to your particular problem, over and above performance anxiety. Once these causes have been dealt with, the issue of performance anxiety and its role in continuing the problem should be addressed. That is the goal of this chapter.

PLAN OF THE PROGRAM

The goal of this self-help program is to enable you to break free of sexual performance anxiety, or self-consciousness and worry about your erection, and the vicious cycle it creates. When a man starts to worry about his sexual performance, and in this instance what is (or will be) happening to his penis, he sort of removes himself from the situation. Instead of focusing his

SEXUAL DYSFUNCTION PROCESS

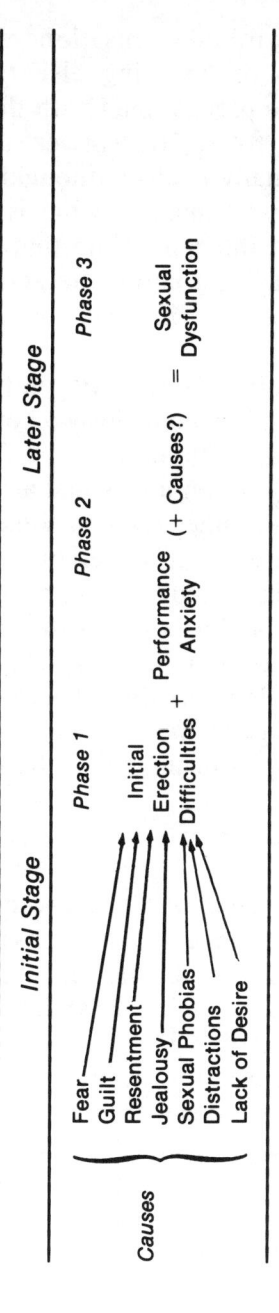

Initial Stage	Later Stage

Phase 1   **Phase 2**   **Phase 3**

Initial
Erection
Difficulties + Performance (+ Causes?) = Sexual
               Anxiety   Dysfunction

Causes {
- Fear
- Guilt
- Resentment
- Jealousy
- Sexual Phobias
- Distractions
- Lack of Desire
}

attention on his own body sensations, his partner's body, her responses to him, or anything else that might be sexually exciting, his mind is preoccupied with thoughts of his penis and what is happening to it. He worries about himself, which is anything but a sexually exciting thought. (Sometimes it can be exciting to let yourself imagine what is going on between you and your partner at the same time that it is happening. In this sense you are fantasizing about the action even as it is taking place. This kind of standing back and observing *is* sexually exciting.)

Overcoming performance anxiety can be accomplished best by eliminating it, that is, by taking away all expectations that you will have to do something with an erection if you get one. That way you will be free to focus on things that are sexually exciting again, that get you aroused, rather than on something like worry, which turns you off. Men who are experiencing erection problems are generally trapped in exactly the opposite pattern: they worry about their penises, and as soon as they do get an erection, they rush to do something with it before it subsides. The desensitization program presented later in this chapter will be your guide to breaking out of this pattern.

A second strategy in dealing with the problem of performance anxiety is to *disprove* your fears. Concerning erection problems, one fear that men commonly have is that an erection, once it is lost, is gone for the night. They approach sexual encounters with a dread of losing an erection. It is a wonder, under such circumstances, that they do get sexually aroused and have erections at all. If they do, they usually become self-conscious, instead of turned on, and their erection subsides. At this point they feel defeated and frustrated. Of course, under these conditions the erection does not return, for they are unable to focus on the kinds of things that will get them aroused again. The exercise in the following section addresses this problem and is intended to demonstrate that sexual arousal, and with it erections, can come and go again and again during a single sexual experience, so long as performance anxiety does not enter the picture to sabotage things.

SEXUAL AROUSAL AND ERECTIONS

Men who experience erection problems tend to share a common fear, that once they lose their erection during a sexual encounter, they will not get it back. Men who are not experiencing erection problems don't usually have this fear. It is no coincidence, furthermore, that men who are experiencing erection problems will not usually get another erection after losing one, whereas men who are not having problems can lose their erection temporarily and get it back later on during a lovemaking session. The difference is that the one group of men worries about themselves, and therefore distracts themselves from sexually exciting stimulation; the others don't get caught up in being self-conscious. Instead, they turn their attention to things that turn them on, like their partner's bodies or the sensations in their own bodies.

Actually, it is not in the least uncommon for a man of any age to lose his erection temporarily once or more during a lovemaking session, especially if it is a long one that involves a number of varied activities and a good deal of give-and-take. This becomes even more likely when a man enters middle age. The fact that his erection may subside does *not* mean, however, that a man has a sexual dysfunction or that he is not turned on by his partner. What is happening is that his level of sexual arousal is varying, and variations in the hardness of his penis follow the variations in his level of arousal. Alhough many sexual activities are pleasant, not all are equally arousing to everyone. The purpose of the following exercise is to demonstrate how variations in your level of sexual arousal can be reflected in variations in the state of your penis.

Exercise 9.1: Getting, Losing, and Regaining Erections
For this exercise you will not need a partner. What you will need is about half an hour of complete privacy. It would be a good idea if you could do this exercise twice or three times on separate days.

Assured that you have privacy, remove your clothes and find a comfortable chair to sit in, or sit up in your bed. Take five or ten minutes to explore your body, but don't touch your genitals. Touch yourself in as many places as you can reach without straining. Use a soft, stroking motion. Notice what the different parts of you feel like and also how they feel when they are touched. You will probably discover places that feel soft, others that seem rougher, and many that feel good when they are touched in a soft, caring manner. This part of the exercise may seem strange at first. It may even make you uncomfortable if you have never paid this sort of attention to your body before. Take your time, however, and keep at it. There is much you can discover about the potential of your own body to give you pleasure.

After you have spent some time exploring your body, proceed to get yourself sexually turned on. In other words, give yourself an erection. To do this you may need to provide yourself with some props. You may, for instance, want to use some hard- or soft-core pornographic material. You may want to use fantasy, either alone or in combination with pornography. You may wish to fantasize about someone you know, or you may want to invent a partner. You will almost certainly have to touch and fondle your own genitals in order to get aroused enough to experience an erection. You may want to experiment with a vibrator. These are available in most department stores. There are different kinds, ranging from those you strap to your hand to ones that you hold. The sort of stimulation you get from a vibrator is very different from the stimulation you get from using your hand alone.

Touch your penis in places and in ways that feel good. Try stroking yourself very gently, then use a firmer touch. Vary the pace of your stroking as well, faster and slower. Notice whether you prefer a light or heavy touch, slow or fast strokes. Notice also which spots on your penis are the most sensitive. At the same time, use your fantasies, magazines, or whatever to help you get turned on.

If you follow this procedure and don't feel especially up-tight about pleasuring yourself, you should be able to bring your penis *to an erect state after a short while. If this doesn't happen, it is almost certainly due to your being distracted, maybe by feelings of guilt or worries about what your partner might be thinking if she knew what you were doing. Whatever the source of your distraction, don't worry. Stop the exercise for today and try again tomorrow. Next time, try to focus in more on your body and move only as fast as you feel comfortable doing.*

Once you have a firm erection, but before you come close to orgasm, **stop.** *Stop your fantasy, close your book if you used one, and stop touching yourself. Just lie back and relax. In a while you will find that your erection will subside.*

Let your erection subside completely *before going on. If it does not subside, chances are you are still giving yourself some stimulation. It could be that you find it difficult to drop your fantasy once you've started it. Whatever the reason, it is important to the exercise that you let your erection subside and the best way to accomplish this is to stop all stimulation and wait.*

After your erection is gone, start pleasuring yourself again. Use the same routine as before, or vary it. If you think you are feeling tense, stop and rest for a moment. This time you don't need to stop stimulating yourself once you have an erection, but you can continue on to orgasm if you like. Some men, however, may want to experiment with losing and regaining their erection twice or even three times before going on to orgasm. Do so if you wish.

This simple exercise can demonstrate to you that it is possible to lose and regain an erection. More than that, it demonstrates how your erection (or lack of it) varies according to how sexually aroused you are. When your attention is focused on things that are sexually exciting (a fantasy, the sensations in your penis, and so on), you get aroused and have an erection; but when you cut yourself off from sources of erotic stimulation, your level of arousal, and your erection, subsides. If this can happen during a self-pleasuring session, it can just as well happen during a sexual encounter.

Chances are that you went through this exercise without feeling tense or self-conscious about your erection. If your experience during sexual encounters is different from your experience when stimulating yourself, the reason has to do with performance anxiety that surfaces when you lose an erection during lovemaking and the fact that by worrying about your performance, you cut yourself off from the kinds of things that contribute to sexual arousal.

UNDERSTANDING DESENSITIZATION

Before you and your partner will be ready to use the procedure described in the following pages to overcome your erection problem, you must teach yourself how to relax. Even though you think you already know how to relax, if you have not yet done so, take the time now to learn the relaxation technique described in chapter 5. When you have had a chance to develop the conditioned relaxation response, you will be in a position to resume this program and get the most out of it. If you go ahead now without first developing the relaxation technique, any trouble with the program will be a sure sign that you need to backtrack.

When psychologists want to help someone overcome anxiety, they often use a procedure called desensitization, discussed earlier in this book. In this process, as you may recall, you begin with a goal in mind, which is to become capable of being in some uncomfortable situation without feeling nervous, and then try to reach that goal through a series of steps. An example might be a man who is afraid of snakes. Assuming that he wants to overcome this fear, his goal would be, say, to be able to stand next to a snake without getting tense. An approach might be to lock him in a room with a snake and hope that he gets used to it, what might be called the "one-jump" approach to overcoming anxiety. A second approach would be to break down the goal—of standing beside a snake—into a series of steps, for example, looking at a picture of a snake, seeing a snake in a cage across the room, and so forth. The one-step-at-a-time approach is used in desensitization.

A second part of the desensitization process involves the relaxation technique, which is used to overcome nervous tension as you move through the steps of the desensitization procedure. To "desensitize" an individual, we would not only want him or her to progress one step at a time, but we would also teach the relaxation technique and encourage the individual to use it at any tense point in the procedure.

The difference between the one-jump and the desensitization approaches in overcoming discomfort is illustrated in the diagrams that follow.

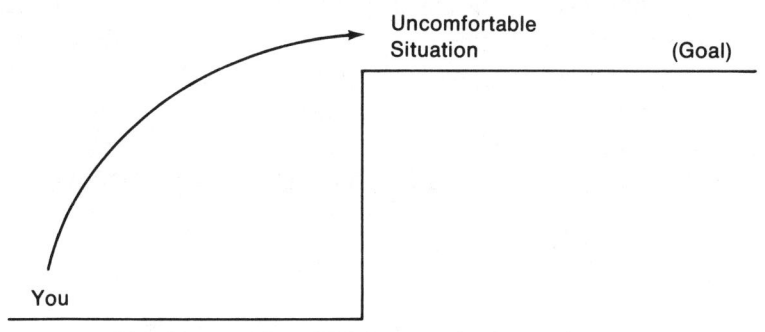

THE ONE-JUMP APPROACH TO OVERCOMING ANXIETY

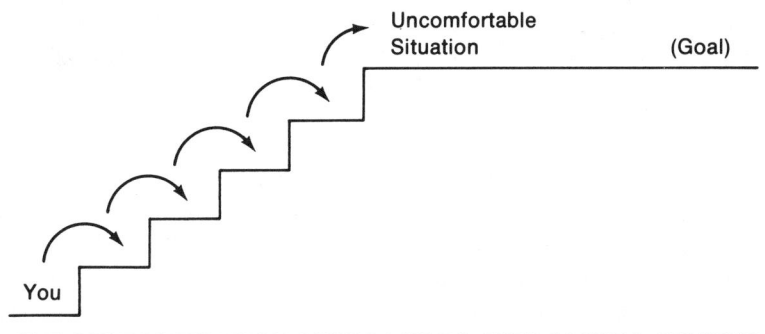

THE DESENSITIZATION APPROACH TO OVERCOMING ANXIETY

There are two major differences between the one-jump and the desensitization approaches. First, the desensitization process takes longer, and therefore requires more patience. Second, the desensitization approach often works; the one-jump approach seldom works.

Your goal in this program is to be able to have erections during your sexual encounters more often than you have been and/or to maintain those erections long enough to have intercourse when you want to. The factor that complicates things—that interferes with your ability to have erections—is performance anxiety. Because of this anxiety, a sexual encounter is for you an "uncomfortable situation," just as being in a room with a snake is an uncomfortable situation for the man in the example. For you to overcome your anxiety effectively, you and your partner together should use the desensitization procedure described here. Again, the first step is for you to develop a way of relaxing yourself that you can apply as need be. The second part is to break down your goal into a series of steps. Then, third, you and your partner can follow this stepwise approach and *rebuild* your sexual relationship *without* performance anxiety.

DESENSITIZATION PROCEDURE FOR ERECTION PROBLEMS

This procedure, or program, consists of seven steps. Read the instructions for Step 1 with your partner before beginning.

Step 1

Arrange two or more evenings in which you and your partner give each other a sensual massage (described in chapter 6, Exercise 6.3). When doing these initial massages, follow the instructions carefully, but it is very important that you observe the following restrictions:

1. Do *not* touch each others' breasts or genitals.
2. If you get an erection at any time during one of these sessions, do *nothing* with it. Do *not* attempt to have intercourse. Do *not* allow your partner to stimulate your penis with her hands, her mouth, or a vibrator.

Take as long as you like for the massage sessions, but at least one full hour each time. Make the setting comfortable and romantic. Get yourselves a vibrator to play with. Without watching the clock, try to spend about as much time receiving (being massaged) as giving (massaging your partner). Finally, and most importantly, be sure to use the relaxation technique to relax yourself if and when you become tense during a session.

These sensual massage sessions will provide you and your partner with an excellent opportunity to develop your sexual communication skills at the same time that you discover more about each other on a physical level. You can begin by making it a point to tell your partner what feels good and what parts of her body please you most. Additional exercises that may be useful in improving sexual communication are found in chapter 3.

The two restrictions placed on you and your partner at this stage of the program may be frustrating at times. If you have not been experiencing erections, but do so during a sensual massage, you will no doubt be tempted to make use of it. Although there is no telling for sure that this won't work, it is risky at this point and may lead to disappointment. At this early stage of the program, you are very likely to become self-conscious when you try to move quickly to intercourse (that is, your attention will probably shift from something that is turning you on to worrying about your penis), with the result that your arousal, and your erection, will subside.

The purpose of the sensual massage is to give and get pleasure and to explore each other in new ways, and the restrictions are intended to prevent you from experiencing performance anxiety. This is a critical step. If you break the restrictions, or believe in your own mind that you would not observe them if you did get an erection, you will probably *not* be able to get away from being self-conscious during your sessions and you may not get an erection at all. It is, therefore, very important that you and your partner both observe the restrictions and follow the instructions as they are laid out. If you can do that, you will be free to enjoy each other during your sessions without worrying about what might happen next.

If your partner finds herself getting highly aroused and would like you to stimulate her further than the instructions in Exercise 6.3 call for, you may bring her to orgasm using your hands, mouth, a vibrator, or whatever, *after* you have finished the massage. If you feel turned on, you can bring yourself to orgasm, alone or with your partner present.

Do not proceed to Step 2 until you are able to have *at least two* sensual massages as described without getting tense. If you have the time, you can do one massage a night and may want to do three or four before moving on.

Step 2

Arrange to have at least two more sensual massages, only this time you may include each others' breasts and genitals as part of them. In other words, follow all the instructions as they are written in Exercise 6.3. Again, make sure that giving and getting are equal priorities for the two of you. You may also want to begin varying your routine a little, rather than repeating the exact one every time. The most important point to observe at this stage of the program, however, is that while you may include breasts and genitals in the massage, do not focus *exclusively* on these areas. Instead, include breasts and genitals as part of an overall massage. Be sure, in addition, to apply the relaxation technique as necessary to let go of tension when you discover it.

By this time, you probably will enjoy your massage sessions very much. If not, perhaps you need to do some work in the area of communication (see chapter 3). Briefly, what you need to do is to tell each other what feels best and what you want, as well as what you don't like or want. You also need to give each other some guidance in pleasuring each other.

If you get an erection during these massages, again do nothing about it. Do not go on to intercourse or have your partner stimulate you to orgasm. If your partner wants this for herself, feel free to pleasure her in any way that you like except with your penis.

During one or more of your Step 2 massages, you may experience at least a partial erection, if only temporarily. This is because, instead of thinking about your penis and what is going to happen to it, your attention will be on things that are sexually exciting, like the sensations in your body or the way your partner looks.

If you do get an erection and feel very turned on during a massage, you can again stimulate yourself to orgasm using your hand and/or a vibrator. Your partner might enjoy watching you, and you might find that it turns you on more to have her there. Also, by watching you stimulate yourself, your partner can learn a lot about how to please you. You may then want to ask her to enjoy herself while you watch.

Should you find yourself often getting tense during the Step 2 massages, and if using the relaxation technique does not seem to help, go back to Step 1 and do a couple of massages that do not include breasts and genitals. Then try Step 2 again.

Continue the sensual massage (including breasts and genitals) until you can do them without feeling up-tight and until you find them at least a little sexually arousing. When these two conditions are being satisfied by your sessions, you will begin to experience erections, if only temporarily, during at least some of your sessions. More likely, you will find them much more exciting than that and will have to resist the temptation to break the intercourse restriction.

Step 3

If you have faithfully followed the previous steps in this program, you now have experienced erections during some of your sensual massages. They may be only partial erections (not as firm as they can be), and they may not last long. That's okay. It is difficult, remember, to break away from a strong habit of self-consciousness and worry, and slow but steady progress is nothing to sneeze at.

The main goal of these sessions until now has been to restart your sexual relationship without performance anxiety entering the picture, or at least to minimize it. These sessions also enable you to learn more about each other and to develop your ability to communicate in bed. If you can do them now without getting up-tight, if you find yourself enjoying them and getting turned on, you can consider yourselves to be doing very well. You are now ready to take another step.

Have two more sensual massage sessions, but this time feel free to try getting each other turned on purposely after a while. Your only restriction is that you still do *not* try to insert your penis into your partner, or attempt intercourse.

Continue to arrange your sessions in ways that are romantic and unhurried. Continue to place as much importance on giving pleasure to each other as you do on getting pleasure for yourselves. Include touching and/or licking of breasts, genitals, and other erogenous zones you may have discovered as part, but not all, of the session. Talk to each other, making sure especially that the other person knows what feels good.

Begin now to make a purposeful effort to vary your routine. For example, start your massage with the feet instead of at the head, start out lying on your back instead of on your stomach, or try massaging each other at the same time. You can also try stimulating yourself while the other person watches. This can be a big turn-on for both of you. If you have not as yet done so, now would be a good time to experiment with a vibrator. Use it on yourselves as well as on each other. Use it briefly at first, and not too intensely on your genitals until you have some time to get used to it. As a source of variety in your sexual relationship, vibrators can be a lot of fun. Or you might, as another way of varying your routine, want to try taking a shower or a bath together, either before or after your massage.

Finally, you might enjoy using different kinds of massage oils, including some that are scented and flavored.

When your partner is touching you to get you turned on, tell her what feels good and guide her, by taking her hand in yours or by showing her by touching yourself, what you like best. Ask her to do likewise when you are touching her. Don't lie still and silent; move around and make noise, even if it seems strange at first.

If at any point you find yourself being self-conscious and worrying about your erection, shift your attention to something more exciting. If you find that your body is tense or that your breathing is constricted, pause to apply the relaxation technique, then proceed.

If the above part of the session goes well, meaning that you are not overly self-conscious and that you or your partner gets turned on, you will experience an erection. This might not happen during every session, but when it does happen, stop touching each other for a while and just lie together quietly. Be still, clear your mind of thoughts, and relax until your erection subsides. When your erection has gone down completely, not before, resume your sensual massage. After a while, ask your partner to stimulate you to erection a second time. You can also ask her to continue stimulating you to the point of orgasm, if you like, and you can do the same for her, before or after your own climax. Do *not* attempt to insert your penis into your partner's vagina at any time during these sessions.

If, during any one of the above sessions, you do not get an erection, or if it subsides and does not return, try again another time. Don't get upset. Remember, you can't expect your sexual performance to be the same each and every time you go to bed, nor can you expect your performance anxiety to disappear all at once. But if the same sort of thing begins to happen consistently—you either don't get or don't keep an erection—return to Step 2.

Following the above instructions may require some patience and self-control on both your parts by now. Having a partner who is interested enough in you and your relationship to follow through with this program is something that deserves appreciation. No doubt it is difficult for both of you at times to follow instructions and heed the restrictions. By doing just that, however, you are maximizing your chances for success. If you are responding as described, you have come a long way by now and should be aware that your sexual performance has already changed substantially. You may still not get an erection during each and every sexual encounter, but that is to be expected. Don't worry too much about any one session. Instead, try to maintain a perspective on yourself and your overall sexual performance over time.

In many ways your lovemaking sessions may already be much more satisfying to you now than they used to be, and this may have a beneficial effect on your relationship in general. Despite occasional frustrations, couples often report a great deal of closeness—a sense of intimacy—as they work together on programs such as this. Don't, however, expect yourselves to be saints. One or the other of you, and sometimes both may lose patience once in a while or give in to feelings of frustration. That is only human. What is more important than perfection is being able to get back together again, either later that same day or the next day, and pick up on the program where you left off. Don't make the mistake of thinking that neither of you should have emotional reactions to this program. It is for sure that you will, and it is much better that you expect this and feel free to express your feelings. If you don't, chances are that these feelings will build up until they surface in other ways, or perhaps in an explosion, which can be destructive to your progress and your relationship. Expressing yourselves and accepting the other's rights to feelings of any kind can be an effective way of preventing such negative things.

When you are able to have two (not necessarily consecutive) sessions like those described above, which include you being stimulated to a point of high arousal twice (followed perhaps by an orgasm), congratulate yourselves, treat yourselves to a good dinner, and proceed to Step 4. Do not, however, jump ahead until you are able to have a minimum of two sessions like this.

Step 4

Continue your sessions as you have been, including genital touching. Feel free to experiment more with your routine and with different ways of pleasing each other. By now you should be enjoying these sessions without feeling a great deal of tension and without much self-consciousness, but you can always use the relaxation technique, as well as the technique of refocusing your attention on something exciting, when you find yourself thinking about what is going to happen to your penis.

If you do not happen to experience an erection during one session, enjoy the time you have together, please each other, and stop for that day or evening. Don't let the state of your penis (erect or nonerect) dictate whether or not a sexual encounter continues or ends, much less whether you enjoy it or not. There are, you will recall, many different reasons why you might not have an erection on any one night, including fatigue, distractions, and so on. You will only be hurting yourself if you overreact and start experiencing a lot of performance anxiety again.

If you do experience an erection some time during the session, and if it either stays with you or subsides and returns, lie on your back and ask your partner to get on top of you, that is, to straddle you. Let her stroke your body, including your genitals, for a while from that position. You can also touch her at first, but after a while you should lie back and just focus on the feelings in your body as your partner touches you. Then, when you feel ready, ask her to move up and insert your penis into her vagina.

Once your penis is contained within your partner's vagina, let the two of you remain fairly still for a minute or so. Focus in on the sensations in your genitals and on your breathing. Let your breathing be free, deep, and easy. After a while, you and your partner can begin to move, slowly. Pump and thrust together, but slowly and easily. Do not pump hard or continue pumping to the point of orgasm. After about a minute of slow thrusting, stop and pull your penis out from your partner's vagina. At this point you can stimulate each other to orgasm, using hands, mouths, vibrators, or whatever you like, except your penis.

If your erection subsides after your penis has been inserted into your partner's vagina, stop moving and lie still. Let your penis remain in her vagina even as your erection subsides. Check your body for tension and use the relaxation technique as needed. Let your partner sit on you, with your penis inside of her, for five minutes while she strokes your body, and concentrate on the way her touch feels. After five minutes, pull your penis out and continue your session, starting with nongenital caressing and massage. If and when you feel relaxed again, try some more genital caressing. Don't worry if you do not get an erection this time—just lie back and enjoy the sensations coming from your genitals. If you do get another erection, you can ask your partner to stimulate you to orgasm, but don't try inserting your penis into her again during this session. Feel free to pleasure your partner to orgasm as many times as she would like in any way other than with your penis.

Step 4 again requires a certain amount of patience and self-control. You and your partner both may want to continue once you have an erection and are inside of her. While this may work out for you, it is still a bit risky at this point, since you may become self-conscious, worry, and defeat yourself. If you do this, you will at least come out of such an experience with a clearer understanding of what you shouldn't do if you want to stay turned on.

When you have had two successful sessions like the above (meaning that you can insert your erect penis into your partner's vagina for a couple of minutes), proceed to Step 5.

Step 5

The sessions you will have now are very similar to those in Step 4, with one difference: to overcome your fear of losing your erection and not getting it back, it would be helpful if your partner could stimulate you to erection and if you could insert your penis into her, *twice*. That is, in these sessions you should repeat the insertion and slow thrusting part of Step 4 a second time. In between, you should lose your erection temporarily.

As you did in Step 4, if and when you feel relaxed and ready, lie on your back and ask your partner to straddle you. Let her caress your body and your genitals, using her hands, her mouth, or a vibrator. If you get an erection, insert it into her vagina and do some slow, easy pumping and thrusting together for a minute or two. Then remove your penis and ask your partner to lie down beside you. Don't touch each other, and try to clear your mind of sexually exciting thoughts. Relax, and wait for your erection to subside. If this doesn't happen, the reason is that you are getting turned on by something. Try to turn it off, whatever it is, temporarily.

When your erection has subsided, begin to caress each other's bodies, including each other's genitals, in order to get sexually aroused a second time. This may not take much time, but then again it might. Take as much time as you need. There is no reason to hurry or to expect your penis to get erect in a certain amount of time. If you do get a second erection, and if your partner is also feeling turned on, insert your penis into her, with her on top, a second time. Again, do some slow thrusting for a few minutes and then withdraw your penis. Finish the session by bringing each other to orgasm, but *not* by intercourse.

When you are able to do the above once, proceed to Step 6.

Step 6

Continue arranging your lovemaking/massage sessions as you have been, experimenting in any ways you like. When you feel sexually aroused and have an erection, let your partner straddle you and insert your penis into her. Begin moving together, slowly at first, pumping and thrusting. Try to develop some rhythm together. Experiment with using your hands to stimulate each other's genitals at the same time that you thrust. Do this for a few minutes, then, after lying still for a minute or so, begin to move again. Continue with this stop-start pattern for as long as you maintain your erection. Gradually let yourselves pump faster and longer. If one or both of you eventually reaches orgasm this way, fine. If you don't, finish off your session when you are ready by bringing each other to orgasm in some other way.

One important point to keep in mind is to try to build up both the intensity and duration of your thrusting and pumping gradually and to include some pauses—times when you stop moving and touching for a minute or so and are relatively still together. You may find that you sometimes lose your erection. As before, the thing to do at such times is to pause. Let your penis stay inside of your partner. Use the relaxation technique to relax any parts of you that seem especially tense. Let your breathing become free and easy. Then touch each other again. Pay attention, not just to your penis, but to other parts of your body and the sensations from them when you are caressed.

If you happen to get turned on and have a second erection, and if your partner is also aroused, ask her to get on top of you, penetrate her, and move together again. You may want to try stimulating her genitals and breasts with your fingers or a vibrator while you are thrusting, and you may even want to bring her to orgasm this way. Your own arousal, meanwhile, may be heightened if she touches your breasts and genitals while you thrust inside of her. She can, for instance, reach behind her and hold or stroke your testicles or squeeze your penis between her fingers.

There may be times when your erection subsides and does not return during these sessions. Hopefully, by now you are past the point of feeling panic about this sort of thing, and you should be able to enjoy the sessions together without the need for an erect penis each and every time.

Try the above sort of session three or four times, and then move on to Step 7.

Step 7

This is the last step in the desensitization program. By using the stop-start procedure described in Step 6, you have gradually built up the intensity and duration of thrusting with your penis inside of your partner's vagina. You may even have been able to reach orgasm in the woman-on-top position. What you need to do now is to experiment with varying your positions. Men do not find all positions equally stimulating (for instance, some cannot reach orgasm in the woman-on-top position), and you need to try out different ones to discover which you like best.

Continue for a while to penetrate your partner, at least initially, with her on top of you, and do some thrusting for a while in this position. After a while, you can try moving to a side-by-side position. You may have to pull out and re-enter in order to shift positions, but you both may find it fun to try to shift without having to pull out. After thrusting together in the side-by-side position for a while, shift again, this time so that you are in the man-on-top position. Continue to use the stop-start procedure, pumping and thrusting slowly at first, for a minute or so, and then pausing before thrusting some more. Gradually let yourself pump and thrust more intensely and longer, until you are able to reach orgasm in a position that is comfortable and sexually arousing for both of you.

If you have proceeded as directed in the desensitization program, your sexual performance will be much different today than it was when you began it. You may still not get an erection during each and every sexual encounter, and you may still sometimes have the experience of losing and not getting a second (or third) erection before reaching orgasm. However, things generally should be much different for you now. The cycle created by self-consciousness and worry over your erection should largely be broken, and your experimentation with sensual massage will probably have changed the nature of your sexual relationship, hopefully in the direction of a greater sense of fulfillment for each of you. Moreover, you can expect things to continue to change as far as your sexual relationship and performance are concerned, and in your relationship in general. At this point you might wish to read or reread chapter 3 (Enhancing Your Sexual Relationship) together, trying out the exercises described there. They aim at furthering the richness of your sexual relationship and increasing the personal fulfillment you can derive from it.

The key to success in this program, once more, is patience and persistence. If things at one step do not go as described right away, continue to work on them for a while. Don't let yourself despair; this will only make matters worse and is not called for. If you do find yourself getting upset because of what is happening when you work on a particular step, back up a step or even two steps. Also, you may want to have occasional sessions that include *only* a sensual massage. These sorts of breaks from the program can be very helpful as well as enjoyable.

If you and your partner feel that you have given the program an honest try, but it does not seem to be working, consider consulting a professional sex therapist. This person should be a licensed psychologist, psychiatrist, or psychiatric social worker who is, first of all, a trained counselor and who has, *in addition to* this basic training, received special training in sex counseling. Such a person may be able to help you identify whatever factor is interfering with your progress and suggest some ways of freeing you. Tell this person about the things you have tried to do to help yourself and show him or her this book. Then follow the advice you get.

BACKSLIDING AND WHAT TO DO ABOUT IT

By the term *backsliding,* we mean a setback, a recurrence of your erection problem. You might consider yourself to be backsliding when you notice a steady decline in your sexual performance over time. This would mean having more and more sexual experiences in which you either don't get an erection, or lose your erection and don't get it back before reaching orgasm. If this happens, you will need to consider what to do about it.

Backsliding is a very different matter than occasional difficulties with getting, or keeping, an erection. Since you are not a sexual machine, you should not expect yourself to perform like one. You can expect yourself to have sexual experiences occasionally during which you don't get an erection, or you lose one and don't get it back. This can be the result of any one of a number of complications. It can also be the result of simple fatigue, too much alcohol, or a temporary depression. None of these effects needs to be more than temporary, and your erection difficulties will pass when they are no longer active.

You should realistically expect your own sexual performance to vary over time. Part of this normal variation may include sexual experiences in which you are exceptionally aroused and able to keep an erection for a long time, or get another erection very soon after reaching orgasm. And, this variation will include times when you don't seem to be able to get highly aroused or maintain your arousal. The one thing to avoid at such times is setting up a performance anxiety cycle in which you start to worry about your sexual performance, become self-conscious, and end up creating a sexual dysfunction.

The first, and perhaps most important, thing you can do to avoid getting into a performance anxiety cycle is to not jump to the conclusion that you are backsliding simply because you have an experience in which you don't get or keep your erection, or even because you have such an experience every so often. Accepting these experiences as a normal part of your sexuality will help you to avoid unnecessary worry.

A second thing you can do is to learn to *adjust* to the normal variations in your sexual performance. In short, you and your partner can become more flexible in terms of your sexual relationship (see chapter 3). If you don't get an erection, don't end your lovemaking there. Spend your time together doing things that are pleasing and exciting, but which don't require an erection (which is just about anything except intercourse). By abandoning your lovemaking solely because you don't have an erection, you are placing an artificial limitation on your sexual relationship. That limitation does not need to be there. It is frustrating, both to you and your partner, and you can do without it simply by not allowing yourself to be ruled by the state of your penis.

A third thing you can do is to use the relaxation technique to relax yourself if and when you are having difficulties. After you have done this, see if you can shift the focus of your session, at least temporarily, away from activities that require an erect penis toward ones that do not, for example, a sensual massage. Focus your attention on your partner's body when you touch her and on your own body when she touches you. If you find your mind wandering to other thoughts, switch your attention back to yourself and your partner and what is happening at the moment. Enjoy what is happening without worrying about what is going to happen.

A fourth thing you might consider when you are in a sexual situation and find it difficult to get or stay aroused is to *take a break* from lovemaking and do something else together for a while. Some activities that different men have tried, and which have worked well for them, include taking a bath or shower together; lying together, either quietly or talking; reading to each other from a sexy or romantic novel or magazine; taking a walk together; playing tag or hide-and-seek in the nude; taking a swim; feeding each other; listening to music; looking at old photo albums; looking through magazines like *Playboy;* making a fire in the fireplace and lying in front of it together; playing strip poker; playing tennis; and so on. These are only a few of the possibilities, but they should give you an idea. What all of these different activities have in common is that they are things that partners can do together and that can be fun and exciting or relaxing. Obviously, not everything in this list is likely to appeal to you. Hopefully, however, the two of you can think of some things that would be pleasing.

If you feel that you are experiencing more than occasional difficulties and that your problems are becoming more frequent over time, it would be in your interest to take some action to curtail this backsliding. You need to reevaluate things, and rereading chapters 8 and 9 is a good place to begin. It would be helpful if you could come to some understanding of just what type of complication may be responsible for your current difficulties, since to some degree different complications call for different solutions. Consider the following two instances:

> At the time he initially saw me, Mr. A was single but moving toward a steady relationship with Ms. B. He had been divorced for about a year and a half and had known Ms. B for a few months. Although during his marriage he had seldom experienced sexual difficulties, since his divorce Mr. A had been having problems both in getting and keeping erections. This was true in his relationship with Ms. B, as well as in all the other relationships he had had since his separation.
>
> The origins of Mr. A's sexual problem had to do with his divorce, which was initiated by his wife of twenty years. A shy man, he liked being married and felt uncomfortable in the singles scene. Also, to make matters even more difficult for him, people in general had changed in some ways during those twenty years that he had been married. Single women, who were now much more forward with their sexual interests, scared him. He suffered, as well, from mixed feelings about women as a result of his wife's rejection. Each of these factors—his personality, changing sexual norms, and feeling burned by the divorce—contributed something to his difficulties in getting and staying aroused during sexual encounters.
>
> In Mr. A's case, his difficulties led in turn to a performance anxiety cycle. He became self-conscious and worried in bed, and even before going to bed he would fear that he was going to "fail." This naturally made the erection problem a self-fulfilling prophecy. Later on, as his relationship with Ms. B developed, but his sexual performance did not change, she expressed a desire to work with him to overcome the problem. When he saw me, Mr. A's erection problem was being maintained mainly by performance anxiety. By following a program like the one in this chapter, and with the help of Ms. B, he was able to overcome the problem in a few weeks.

As I found out when Mr. A called me several months later, shortly after he had completed his program, he had asked Ms. B to move in with him and she had accepted. Their relationship in turn became closer and more rewarding. Mr. A was very pleased. However, within a few months he was again experiencing, on a regular basis, problems getting an erection.

This time the difficulties did not seem to be linked mainly to performance anxiety. Instead, it appeared that fear was now the main complicating factor, specifically a fear of pregnancy. Ms. B, who was ten years younger than Mr. A and who had never been married or pregnant, had begun to express a wish to have a child with Mr. A, even out of wedlock. Although in some ways this idea had appeal, by and large the prospect of having a baby worried Mr. A, aged forty-two, more than it excited him. When I suggested that this might be the reason for his current sexual difficulties, he agreed that the idea of Ms. B getting pregnant did cross his mind often, especially when they went to bed. Moreover, he privately feared that she might, on an impulse, see to it that she got her wish by secretly having her IUD (intrauterine device) removed. He confided that he had been afraid to confront Ms. B, either with his real feelings about having a child or with his fears about her removing her contraceptive, for fear that she would leave him.

It must be clear how Mr. A's second sexual problem, his backsliding, had to do with a crisis in his relationship with Ms. B over the issue of pregnancy. Before the sexual problem could be overcome, this crisis, and consequently Mr. A's fear, would have to be confronted and resolved. It was my impression that this crisis would not be an easy one to deal with and that it could well place the relationship at risk. So I recommended that the couple consult a marriage counselor and then return to me if the crisis was resolved but the erection problem continued.

Mr. C was single, in his early thirties. He came to see me with a somewhat unusual story. When he was in his midtwenties, he had become involved with a married woman, Mrs. X, and had fallen in love with her. She was his first sexual partner and treated him caringly but, probably because of guilt feelings combined with fears of getting caught by the husband, Mr. C had trouble getting and keeping erections during their sexual encounters. As he recounted the events, these initial difficulties led in turn to a performance anxiety cycle, which interfered with his sexual performance throughout their relationship. She broke it off after a year, not primarily for sexual reasons, but because she wanted to try to make her marriage work.

By a stroke of luck, Mr. C's second sexual partner turned out to be a woman with whom he felt very relaxed and who, in addition, told him that she wanted to go to bed with him, but did not want to have intercourse with him right away. This request came as a great relief to Mr. C, and he was only too happy to agree. Because he was not concerned about needing an erection, he did experience one during his first sexual encounter with this woman. In fact, after that and until he came to see me, Mr. C rarely experienced problems getting or keeping an erection.

He came to see me because he had, by coincidence, met Mrs. X again, a few months before. She was now divorced and had expressed a clear desire to renew her relationship with Mr. C. He still had strong feelings for her, and so they had resumed dating. The problem was that Mr. C's old erection difficulties returned the first time they went to bed, and they had stayed with him ever since.

In talking with me, Mr. C revealed a pattern of behavior that I recognized immediately as a performance anxiety cycle. First he described how, from the moment he had met her again, he had been bothered by unpleasant memories of his past sexual performance with Mrs. X. Then, starting with the first sexual encounter after their reunion, he was self-conscious, worrying that he would not get an erection. Sure enough, he did not get one. Since then they had gone to bed many times, but his performance was seldom what he wanted it to be, or what he knew it could be from his experience with other women. Understandably, he was very upset.

In the case of Mr. C, performance anxiety was responsible for the maintenance of his earlier difficulties (although they were initially caused by guilt and fear); it seemed to be the actual cause, furthermore, of his second round of trouble. It is perhaps a bit ironic that his anxieties were triggered, in both instances, by the same woman, but such things do happen. In this case I recommended that the couple use a desensitization program like the one in this chapter. Mrs. X was hesitant at first, but later she was willing to work with Mr. C under the agreement that doing so would not imply any permanent commitment to him on her part. This understanding was important because she did not, at that time, feel ready to consider an exclusive or committed relationship. They worked well together, as it turned out, and Mr. C's problem was resolved.

The point was made in chapter 8 that an erection problem can have any number of causes, and the above examples illustrate this. Of course, the most common single cause of continuing erection problems is performance anxiety, for which the desensitization program in this chapter is useful.

When and if you find yourself backsliding, consider the alternatives discussed in chapter 8 to determine its basis. If the problem seems to have something to do with your relationship, the only effective way to resolve it must begin by confronting the issue with your partner. Hopefully, together you will be able to work it out. If you conclude that the most likely explanation for the backsliding is some factor within you—for instance, guilt—or within the situation—for example, distractions—you would do well to follow the guidelines in chapter 8 for dealing with it. If you feel that you have fallen into a performance anxiety cycle, which usually happens after you have experienced some initial difficulties caused by something else, going back to the program outlined in this chapter will be the most effective way to deal with it. You may need to start at Step 1 again, or you may be able to start at Step 2 or higher. Wherever you start, you will know whether it was the right place or not by how it turns out. If things do not go well, back up a step or two.

Falling into a performance anxiety cycle and having your sexual performance backslide are never pleasant experiences, but neither should they be causes for despair. Such things happen sometimes, even when you think you have things under control. It is very difficult for a man to completely avoid being self-conscious during a sexual encounter because of the traditional male sexual script he is taught. To a greater or lesser extent, every man wants to be a good lover and so tends to give himself grades for his sexual performance. This means being self-conscious and worrying at times about how things are going. It should come as no surprise to anyone, then, that men can fall into performance anxiety cycles and experience erection problems more than once in their lives.

The more you can get away from the male sexual script, and stop watching and judging yourself in bed, the better off you will be. However, equally important is to keep in mind that when you do experience backsliding there are effective ways of dealing with it. If you need to deal with such problems only once in your life, well and good; but if you need to go through a program like this, maybe one, two, three, or even four times, that is okay, too.

A NOTE FOR SINGLE MEN

As we noted earlier, attempting to use the desensitization program in this chapter presents unique problems if you are a single man who doesn't have a steady partner. To begin with, the task of getting a partner who is willing to participate cooperatively in the program is much simpler for men who are either married or living with women than it is for men who do not have one steady sexual partner. Assuming that their relationships are in a good enough state that they can work together for their mutual benefit, men in steady relationships have a distinct advantage.

One problem that single men who begin to experience erection difficulties are likely to face is a growing fear of getting sexually involved with women at all. Because they fear embarrassment, many single men start avoiding women more and more as their sexual problem develops. Sometimes they avoid women altogether, but more often they just avoid getting involved to the point where the possibility of a sexual relationship enters the picture.

In either case, the idea of getting sexually involved with a woman, even though it might be very exciting, generates a lot of concern. Later on, when they decide to try to overcome the problem, these men can get very upset when they learn that in order to deal with the problem they will first have to get sexually involved and take the risk of having sexual difficulties. Many a look of disappointment and worry has crossed the faces of men after telling them that there really is no way to "cure" a sexual problem alone, *before* going to bed with a woman. Sometimes the thought that they will have to risk a sexual "failure" in order to help themselves has been so upsetting that men have rejected help, asking instead for the name of a surgeon who does prosthetic implants. The desire for an instant cure that would enable men to go to bed with a woman and instantly have an erection is understandable, but the truth is that there simply is no such cure.

If you have been avoiding women, the first thing you may need to do, depending on just how far you have gone, is to restart your social life. If you are not dating at all, you must overcome that problem before you can get to the sexual one. This will almost certainly not be an easy thing to do. Men usually experience a great deal of anxiety when they begin to pursue relationships with women after having avoided them for a time. In general, the longer they have avoided women, the harder it is for them to start things again. In trying to deal with this, some have taken the direct method of just approaching women for dates and/or sex, and this sometimes has worked out well. In fact, sometimes (but not often) the men discovered that their old sexual problems had disappeared. Other men prefer to take things a little slower and resume a social life one step at a time. Some guidelines for this approach can be found in chapter 7 in the section on Sexual Shyness. In addition, several of the exercises in chapter 3, in the section on Sexual Communication, may be useful.

Once your social life is moving again, at least to the point where you are actively dating at least one woman, you will soon come to a second crossroads, and that will be when you have an opportunity for sexual contact. I have spent hours talking with men, hassling out the pros and cons of telling a potential lover ahead of time about past sexual experiences and current fears of involvement. As noted earlier, there doesn't seem to be any one best way of handling the situation. At times it seems to have worked out well when a man has disclosed things beforehand. If the circumstances are right, this self-disclosure can be a great relief and can draw a man and woman closer together. However, if you contemplate doing this, read chapter 7 first and, as a reminder, consider the following guidelines:

It is important that you feel you can trust the woman to whom you choose to make such a disclosure, and trust usually takes some time to develop. You might try sharing some other nonsexual but personal information about yourself first and see how this is received, as well as how you feel about sharing it, before you talk about sex.

Sharing information about your sexual history and concerns with a woman you have just met is, as a general rule, a risky thing to do, since you don't usually know the woman well enough to anticipate how she will react. You might not even be sure yet if she is sexually attracted to you, so talking about what might happen in bed could be considered premature or even rude.

If you meet a woman who seems to be mainly interested in having one sexual encounter, rather than a relationship, with you, trying to talk about sexual fears may not work out well. She may simply not be interested enough to get that involved.

Being able to talk to a woman about your sexual concerns may make you feel better, but it is no guarantee that you won't

> experience difficulties during a sexual encounter with her. Similarly, just because she seems concerned and sympathetic does not mean that a woman will know how to help you (or necessarily want to).
>
> Some women may be sympathetic to you, yet they may decide not to pursue a sexual relationship after you talk to them about your sexual concerns. They may, for instance, feel that you expect them to help you when they are not sure they want to get that involved with you at the time. Or they may have sexual concerns of their own and be looking for a man who could help them.
>
> You can't expect every woman to have a sympathetic attitude. Some may reject you, sometimes in a not particularly caring way, if you tell them you have had sexual difficulties. Although this does not seem to be a common reaction from women, it does happen occasionally, and you should be prepared for it. If it does happen to you, you may be more cautious the next time, but it doesn't mean you were a fool to try it in the first place.

The alternative to disclosing your past sexual problems and your current fear of failure ahead of time is to keep it to yourself and let things happen as they will. This means going ahead with a sexual encounter when it seems right to you. You may be surprised and not have any sexual difficulties, but most likely you will. You can, if you feel that the woman you are with is interested, talk to her about it afterward, in as much or as little detail as you feel comfortable doing.

Not disclosing your sexual concerns in advance also gives you a degree of freedom in a new relationship, in that you don't have to worry about *when* to talk about "it." By deciding that it is all right just to go ahead and enjoy yourself, you can be freer to enjoy the relationship without having to worry about when you should make the big announcement.

Whether you decide to disclose your sexual concerns to a potential lover or keep them to yourself, pay some attention to the timing of a first encounter with a new lover. Try to be sure that the situation is right for *you,* as well as for her. Don't defeat yourself by going to bed with a woman who is interested in you, but to whom you are not attracted, and expect yourself to get highly aroused. If you would prefer to build something of a relationship before moving into sex, assert yourself and set limits that will be good for you. Last, try to get beyond your performance anxiety, at least far enough to be able to enjoy yourself and the woman you are with, even if you don't get an erection. Do not let your sexual encounter stand or fall on the issue of your erection.

The third issue that single men must face is that of finding a woman who is interested enough in them and their relationship to go through the desensitization program as a partner. Many men feel that asking a woman to help them in this way is asking a lot, and in one sense they are right. It is asking a woman to invest something in you and your relationship together, and if she feels that she is not likely to get very much in return, it is an unreasonable request, and she will probably turn you down. The question is, of course, what is a "reasonable return"? Surely, going through the program together implies something about your feelings for one another. But does it imply a permanent or deep commitment to the relationship on your part, her part, or both? Again, there is no simple answer. There are, however, some additional guidelines to offer, gathered from my experience in working with single men.

> *Do not waste your time looking for a woman to whom you can pay money for going through the desensitization program with you. The experiences of sex therapy centers that have used paid "surrogates" have not, by and large, been good. Women who are being paid for their services may be successful in giving a man an erection. This is partly because the situation itself (being with a bought woman) is exciting to many men and partly because paid women are willing to forget about themselves and work on you for their money. The problems enter in later on, when you want to have a sexual relationship with a woman who is not concerned only with pleasing you and earning money. In*

short, your improvement under such circumstances will probably be temporary.

Do not spend your time searching for a potential partner for the desensitization program. Approaching all relationships with this in the back of your mind is likely to ruin the possibilities for other pleasures in those relationships. Men who have spent their time "shopping around" for a woman to help them with their sexual problems report that this approach makes them tense and uncomfortable. Not a few have had rather unpleasant experiences with women who may feel put off and angry when they realize that a man they like is interested in them only as a potential partner for a sex therapy program, as an amateur sex therapist, or both. Rather than shopping for a partner for the program, you should look for women with whom you want to have relationships. If, later on, one of those women is interested in going through the program with you, well and good; if not, you may still want that relationship.

Although it is important that you do not take for granted what you are asking of a woman when you approach her about being your partner in the desensitization program, don't go to the other extreme and think that you are the only one who will get something out of it. The program will require patience and a willingness to tolerate frustration at times. To some extent the planned, stepwise nature of the program is mechanical, and it may make you uncomfortable at first. To a degree it does not permit you to be as free and spontaneous as you both might like to be. On the other hand, unless you let yourself become preoccupied with such feelings, they are likely to fade after a while, at which point your sessions together will, in many ways, be highly pleasurable for **both** *of you. By developing the art of sensual massage, you will both be learning a great deal about each other, including how to give each other pleasure. Don't underestimate the amount of enjoyment you can derive from these sessions and how much you will be able to please your partner at the same time you work toward overcoming your erection problem.*

If you are single and have several actual or potential sexual partners, you need to think about whether you want to ask one, or more than one, of those women to work with you on the desensitization program. Although not all men do this, it is recommended that you go through the program with just *one* partner. Trying to move through a structured program such as this with more than one woman at a time creates a lot of problems. For example, it does not seem reasonable to think in terms of doing one step with one partner and the next step with a different partner. An important part of the procedure is learning to relax as you go through the steps, and it is not likely that you will be able to stay relaxed when you change partners. Then, too, having to explain to a woman that you have already done Step 1 and Step 2 with one woman, and need her for Step 3, is not a situation to be relished by most men. Another difficulty can arise if you try to move through the whole program with more than one woman at the same time. Even if you could find the time to do this, it would almost certainly lead to some very awkward situations. What, for instance, do you do if you seem ready to move up a step with one woman but not another?

Assuming that you decide in favor of having just one partner, you will also need to decide what to do about any other sexual relationships you have now or that might develop during the program. Most men seem to feel best putting all other sexual relationships on hold while they work with one particular woman on the program, and for several reasons this seems to be the best choice. Some men, however, seem to do well by limiting only the one sexual relationship (the one with their program partner) and keeping others open. This alternative seems risky, however, since you may continue to experience performance anxiety in the "free" relationships, and this can impede your progress in general.

In attempting to use the desensitization procedure to help yourself overcome your erection problem, you will, as a single man, need to be even more flexible than will a married man.

The fact that your relationship with your partner is probably a less committed one dictates that you be ready and willing to make compromises between your needs and those of your partner. You may not, for instance, be able to start at Step 1. You may not be able to have as many sessions at each step as the program calls for. You may also have to change the procedure here and there to accommodate your partner's needs and preferences. You should try to stick to the program as it is written as best you can, but not at the cost of your partner's good feelings about you and your relationship.

SUMMARY

This chapter presents a program designed specifically to enable you to overcome sexual performance anxiety, which is probably the most common cause of continuing erection difficulties. Once a man has experienced some initial difficulties with erections, whatever the cause, he may become self-conscious about his sexual performance. Worrying about your erection while attempting to make love will not lead to high sexual arousal on your part; therefore, you may not experience an erection, or you may lose it and not get it back. The same thing happens when a man tries to hurry and use his erection quickly, for fear that it will subside. Similarly, panic after losing an initial erection effectively sabotages your chances of regaining it.

The way to deal with the vicious cycle created by sexual performance anxiety is to restart your sexual relationship. This requires the cooperation of two people. With the understanding that you will not attempt to have intercourse, but will focus instead on giving and getting pleasure and on discovering more about each other on a physical level, performance anxiety can be short-circuited. The key to success is to move a step at a time while focusing your attention on what turns you on, rather than being in a hurry and focusing on worrisome things that turn you off.

Although the exercises described here are intended to deal with erection problems in men, the pleasure that can be gotten from them is not one-sided. Women generally find them very enjoyable, and couples experience benefits above and beyond solving an erection problem. Still, it is better to have developed something of a relationship with a woman before asking her to work with you on the program. This may present a problem if you are a single man who does not have a steady sexual partner, or if you have been avoiding women because of your sexual problem. If issues like this can be resolved, however, the chances of the program being helpful are high.

On Our Anniversary

A girl you were
Upping me in flushes.
Still like a stallion
I flare in your musky scent.
A dozen years have turned
You loose, ripening like
A tart, wormed apple.
A woman you are
Upping me
Quieter,
Tender.
ARTHUR DOBRIN

10 learning to delay orgasm

A man's sexual response is not something that remains constant over time, but is something that naturally tends to vary. Evidence of this is found in men's tendencies to reach orgasm more quickly at some times, more slowly at others. In general, the longer it has been since you last experienced orgasm, the more likely you are to reach that point of arousal quickly. For example, if you have neither masturbated nor had a sexual encounter for several days, and then have intercourse, chances are that you will reach orgasm more quickly than if you had a few orgasms during that time. This pattern also holds true for your sexual performance within a single sexual encounter. It will, generally speaking, take longer to reach orgasm a second time, longer still to reach it a third time, and so on.

Aside from the effects of time, men also differ from one another in terms of how long it usually takes them to reach orgasm. That is, some men have a natural tendency to reach orgasm more quickly than others. The Kinsey sex researchers, for instance, found from their surveys that three out of four men reached orgasm within two minutes after starting intercourse. They also found that some men have a natural tendency to reach orgasm within seconds after penetration (or in some cases, even before they can penetrate completely), while others need a lot longer. Some men, in other words, need very little and others need a great deal of the sort of direct stimulation of their penises that intercourse provides in order to climax.

Today, many men with a natural tendency to reach orgasm quickly are prone to look on this as a problem. Indeed, some therapists and researchers go so far as to label it a sexual dysfunction. However, such a label may be inappropriate, since there is no evidence that anything in the nature of a "breakdown" is involved here, for example, in the sense that erection difficulties represent a "breakdown" in sexual performance from its normal pattern. What we are dealing with in the case of premature ejaculation, as the tendency to come quickly is called, is not something abnormal, but rather is a normal tendency that some men would like to change.

If you are a man who would like to be able to delay orgasm more than you presently can, the program in this chapter may be helpful. As a first step, you should take a look at your attitudes toward yourself. Do you regard yourself as "abnormal" because, during a sexual encounter you are prone to reaching orgasm quickly? Do you think you have a sexual dysfunction, meaning a sexual handicap?

If you answered yes to those questions, you probably at least feel tense about sex and may even feel so ashamed that you avoid women for fear of being embarrassed by your "handicap." Many men in your position find themselves in a similar bind. In their own minds, their sexual performance is lacking, so they expect to be rejected or thought less of by women who would go to bed with them. Rather than going through such an experience, they may choose to avoid sex. This, as we know, becomes a vicious cycle, with the "handicap" growing worse and worse in their own minds the longer they avoid women. As a result of this cycle, some men end up positively fearing women. Their situations are made worse, of course, by the isolation that this fear creates. Because they won't risk sexual encounters, they do not have the opportunity to see how women will really react to their "problem."

Actually, that a man comes quickly during a sexual encounter is not in the least unusual. It seems to happen often, especially during the initial stages of a sexual relationship. Also, although the speed with which they reach orgasm may be a major concern of men, it does not seem to be as important to women. Certainly it matters, but for most women a man's overall lovemaking skills and interest in them count a lot more than how quickly he comes. Most important among these "skills" are gentleness and consideration, plus the ability to be affectionate, romantic, and passionate.

Women seem most attracted to men who appreciate them, physically and otherwise, and who show it in the way they make love and treat them in general. Their chief complaints, sexually speaking, are that too many men are preoccupied with intercourse to the exclusion of other sexual activities and are content to end a sexual encounter just as soon as they have climaxed, be that after one minute or twenty. It would be useful for you to keep this in mind, not only because it may relieve you of feeling that the speed with which you reach orgasm is the most important factor in lovemaking, but also because it will point you in the right direction in terms of what women really want in a sexual relationship.

Another concern expressed by men who come quickly is that this tendency will be so frustrating to a woman that she will end their relationship and look elsewhere. Men also frequently believe that unless they can prolong intercourse their partner will not be able to come. This is based, in turn, on a belief that any (and every) woman can come during intercourse, if only it lasts long enough. But this is not true. Not all women report that they are able to reach orgasm through intercourse, no matter how long it lasts; therefore, not all women expect to reach orgasm this way.

Many of them, however, pretend to do so just to please their partner.

What is likely to be frustrating to your partner is not whether she can reach orgasm through intercourse, but whether you are interested and willing enough to bring her to orgasm by *some* means during your sexual encounters, even if that takes awhile.

CONTROLLING YOUR AROUSAL: WHAT TO EXPECT

What seems to lie at the heart of the concern expressed by men whose natural tendency is to reach orgasm quickly is their feeling that they have no control over their level of sexual arousal. As they describe it, it seems to run its own course, no matter what they do. This leaves them feeling helpless and frustrated. They are under the impression that other men, because it takes them longer to come, are more in control of their arousal. But this may not be the case. For instance, can these other men come quickly if they want to? That is doubtful.

Men who tend to reach orgasm more slowly do not appear to possess some natural ability to control their level of arousal. What they have, if anything, is a greater awareness of that level of arousal. They have this, in turn, simply because their arousal increases more slowly. They can, therefore, delay orgasm by doing things that reduce the level of arousal. What they do is to subtract, or cut off, one or more sources of stimulation, which then reduces their arousal. When they want to come, they add on sources of stimulation until they reach that peak of excitement at which they climax. It is in this sense, then, of being able to add or subtract sources of arousal, that these men seem to be able to "control" their own sexual responses. The basis of this, however, is simply that their arousal naturally tends to increase more slowly.

If you look at the issue of delaying orgasm from this perspective, you can see that those men who feel that they come too quickly are at a disadvantage, *not* because they are lacking something (willpower or self-control), but because their natural tendency is for their arousal to build up so quickly that they have less time to monitor or check it. So they have less of an opportunity to do something about it. Their arousal rises so fast, especially after penetration, that there is little time for them to identify, much less cut off, sources of stimulation before the critical point. In addition, whereas other men may be able to "control" their arousal and delay orgasm by subtracting just a little from their sources of stimulation (for instance, thrusting more slowly for a while), the men with faster arousal may need to subtract many, if not all, sources to avert reaching climax.

Despite differences in the rate at which arousal naturally tends to build, most men can, if they practice long enough, learn to increase the awareness of their own level of arousal. They can then learn to delay or accelerate orgasm by developing some skill in subtracting and adding sources of stimulation that contribute to the arousal. Some men whose natural response involves a sharp rise in arousal after penetration may never get to the point of being able to "control" themselves as much as they might want to, but they can almost always learn to increase their ability to delay orgasm more than they currently can.

CHANNELS OF STIMULATION AND SEXUAL AROUSAL

Feeling sexually turned on is a response in you that is determined by a number of factors. One is the extent to which you find your partner, real or imagined, sexually attractive. This is a matter of personal taste and has to do with your personal sexual interest schema, as discussed in chapter 2. Briefly, the more a particular woman fits your personal preferences in terms of what is sexually appealing in appearance and personality, the more turned on to her you will be. A second factor concerns the situation, the particular circumstances you find yourself in when the opportunity for a sexual encounter arises. The more these circumstances appeal to you, the more sexually excited you can get in that situation.

Additional sources of sexual arousal come from the sexual encounter itself. The first has to do with the content of the encounter or, more simply, the sorts of activities you and your partner engage in. People usually find some sexual acts more exciting than others. If you engage in the kinds of activities *you* find exciting, you will be more turned on than you would if your encounter consisted of activities that appealed to you less.

The ways that your partner's body looks, feels, smells, and/or tastes, as well as the way she responds to what you do to her, are other major sources of sexual arousal. In fact, traditionally this has been a greater source of erotic stimulation for men than it has been for women. This is because of the sexual arrangement in our culture that calls for the man to be the more active partner—the doer—in a sexual encounter. The important point to keep in mind is that your partner's body and the way she responds to you are probably an important channel of erotic stimulation for you as a man.

Your own body is, of course, yet another source of erotic stimulation. Your body contains many erogenous zones, areas that lead to a feeling of sexual excitement when they are stroked or caressed. The one erogenous zone men tend to focus on is the glans, or head, of the penis. Women also tend to focus on this one place when they want to get a man turned on in bed. However, it would be a mistake to think that this is the only erogenous zone on a man's body. He can, and will, get turned on by having many other parts of his body caressed, for example, his lips, nipples, ears, and thighs. Women who appreciate the erotic potential of men's bodies can turn them on by caressing them in the right way almost anywhere.

Each of the above sources of erotic stimulation contributes

something to your total sexual arousal. The more you are able to use each of these channels of stimulation, the more turned on you will be, as the diagram below illustrates.

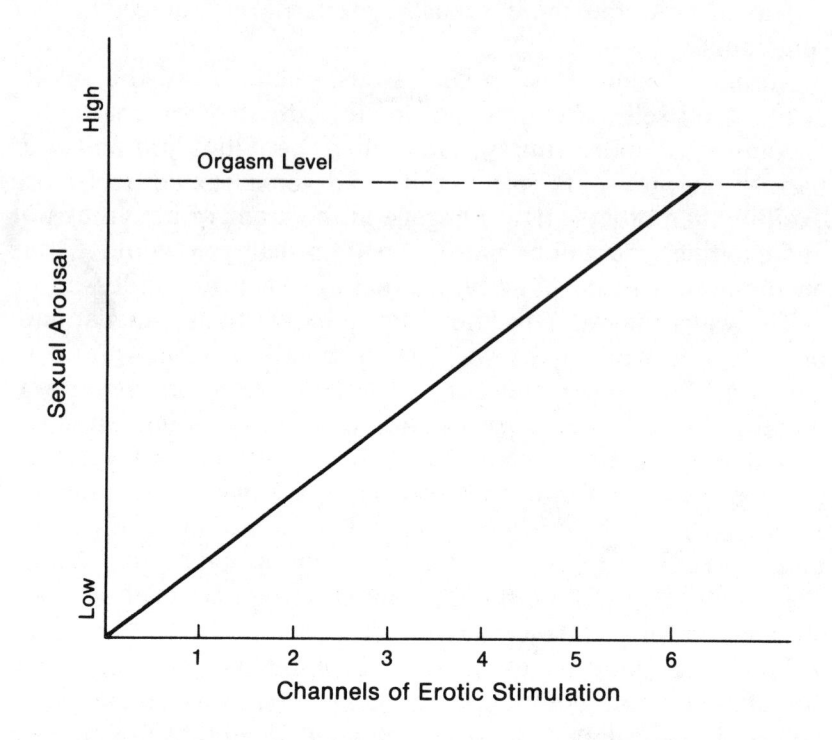

Figure: Sexual Arousal vs. Channels of Erotic Stimulation, showing a linear increase reaching the Orgasm Level at approximately 6 channels.

As the diagram suggests, the man who is able to utilize, say, four separate channels of stimulation is in a position to get more highly aroused than a man who can use only one. It also makes it more likely that his arousal will get high enough for him to reach orgasm. How many he uses depends, of course, on both him and his partner.

Aside from *how many* different channels of stimulation he may use, a man's level of arousal will also depend on *how much* he uses each one. Some men (and/or their partners), for instance, rely almost exclusively on the glans of the penis as a source of erotic stimulation, but they get enough stimulation from this to reach orgasm. Other men may get a lot of stimulation through the penis, but they may also get turned on by looking at their partner's body, watching what she does to them, or fantasizing about a sexually exciting scene. The following exercise illustrates this.

Exercise 10.1: Manipulating Your Arousal

Buy yourself a sexy men's magazine—the kind that has pictures in it—and arrange for half an hour of uninterrupted privacy.

Take your clothes off and lie down on your bed. Look through the pictures in the magazine. Take your time and don't do anything else. After you have looked through the magazine for a while, pay attention to your body. Are you aware of feeling turned on? How would you describe this feeling? Where is the center (or centers) of this feeling located in your body?

Now stroke your penis. At the same time, look at the pictures in the magazine or, if you prefer, close the magazine, close your eyes, and imagine a picture or create a fantasy. You may want to put yourself into your fantasy, imagining for instance that you are making love to one of the women in the pictures, or you may want to imagine yourself watching another man making love to her. Whichever you prefer, just make sure you do it while you are stroking your penis. Do this for a couple of minutes, but try not to bring yourself to orgasm.

After you have stroked yourself and used the magazine (or a fantasy) for a few minutes, stop what you are doing and focus on your body again. How sexually aroused are you now, as compared to when you were just looking through the magazine? Again, how would you describe the feeling of sexual arousal?

Now start to stroke your penis again, but try not *to think about or look at the women in the pictures. Try, in fact, to erase all sexy thoughts from your mind. Close your eyes and stroke your penis, but don't think about anything. Do this for a minute or so.*

The last part of this exercise may be difficult, or even impossible, for you to do. However, if you can do it at all, pay attention to your body again afterward. How turned on are you feeling now?

Finish your self-pleasuring session in any way you like. You may want to bring yourself to orgasm or you may want to invite your partner to join you in bed.

The purpose of this exercise is to demonstrate in a direct way how adding and subtracting channels of stimulation affect your level of sexual arousal. At first, you had essentially one channel operating—the way the women in the pictures looked. You may also have imagined how they might have felt, smelled, or tasted. You may have imagined doing sexually exciting things with them. Whatever, the end result was that you probably did get turned on, in this instance, through psychic stimulation—sights, sounds, smells, and tastes, real or imagined.

In the second phase, you added a second channel of stimulation. This was direct stimulation, having one or more erogenous zones of your body stimulated. In this exercise it was your penis that was directly stimulated by you. By adding this stimulation to what you got from looking at the magazine or fantasizing, you probably were aware that your level of sexual arousal increased.

In the final part of the exercise, you subtracted a channel of stimulation; you were asked to stop looking and/or imagining. If you were able to do this, you probably noticed that your level of arousal decreased. By doing this, you may have also learned one way of reducing your arousal, when and if you want to.

PLAN OF THE PROGRAM

In learning to delay orgasm, the strategy found to be most effective aims at improving your awareness of your own level of sexual arousal. Basically, the procedure involves learning to let your arousal increase slowly (or as slowly as possible) until you are close to the point of orgasm, and then stopping (or minimizing) stimulation temporarily. After your arousal subsides, stimulation is then resumed, until you get to a point of high arousal again. Then it is cut off again. And so on.

As elsewhere in this book, the approach to delaying orgasm will be step-by-step, starting with self-stimulation. We will begin at this point rather than with a partner because self-stimulation is less complicated—there is less distraction when you are alone, so you can focus on yourself and your level of arousal better. Also, when you are stimulating yourself, you have somewhat more control over the channels of stimulation you use, as well as the intensity of any particular one. This, too, will be an advantage in the early stages of the program.

Remember that by learning to become more aware of how sexually excited you are, you can learn to control your arousal to some extent by adding or subtracting sources of stimulation and by varying the intensity of any one channel. This will take some time, however, to learn. The more quickly you are naturally prone to reaching orgasm, the longer it will probably take you to learn to delay it. Expect slow but steady progress. Also, expect that your ability to delay will develop unevenly. Sometimes you will still come quickly, even when your control is getting better. Try not to let this throw you. Remember, this is a natural response on your part that you are trying to change, not something abnormal that you are trying to "cure."

During the later stages of this program, you will need to work with a partner who is willing to cooperate with you to help you learn to delay orgasm. Hopefully, both of you will view this as a desirable goal for your relationship, not just for you as an individual. If you are married or in a steady sexual relationship, talk to your partner about your desire to learn to control orgasm better. Ask her to read this chapter, then discuss it together. Aim at reaching a joint decision about the program—your chances of getting something from your efforts are much better if you can set your goals together and work cooperatively.

You will need a partner to work on the more advanced phases

of the program. Obviously, if you do not have a steady sexual partner, this may be a problem. You can begin the program by yourself since you do not need a partner in the early stages. You should also read the last section in chapter 9, A Note For Single Men, and follow the guidelines there. When you have had a chance to develop a relationship with a woman who you think is interested enough in you and your relationship to participate as your partner in the program, have her read this material. Talk about it, then give her some time to think before asking her to make a decision.

LEARNING TO DELAY ORGASM

This program consists of five steps. Read the instructions for Step 1 completely before starting.

Step 1

To begin the process of learning to delay orgasm, you should develop some skill in monitoring your level of sexual arousal and controlling that level when you are stimulating yourself. To start, make sure that you have about half an hour of privacy. You may wish, in addition, to get some erotic aids — men's magazines, books, and so on. Also—and this is very important—place a clock or watch close at hand where you can see it without having to move around a lot. Take this book with you, too, as well as a pen or pencil, since you will be filling out the Stimulation and Pause Record as you proceed.

Make a note of the time you begin. Write it down on the Stimulation and Pause Record in the column for Session 1, next to Stimulation 1 Start. Following is an example of how this might look.

Session 1

Stimulation 1	Start: *7:35*

Now begin to stimulate yourself in any way that gets you turned on. Stroke yourself and look at your magazines, or create an exciting fantasy in your own mind. Continue to get yourself aroused to a point where you think that you are *close to orgasm*, that is, a level of arousal where you feel that just a little more stimulation will cause you to come. At that point, stop stimulating yourself. Stop stroking yourself, close your magazine, stop fantasizing—stop doing all of the things you have been doing to get yourself turned on. Do not, however, let go of your penis; instead, continue to hold it without stroking it. Look at your watch or clock and make a note of the time. Write down the time on the Stimulation and Pause Record, beside the word Stop. For example:

Session 1

Stimulation 1	Start: 7:35
	Stop: *7:45*

Now, pause. Lie quietly, holding your penis, just long enough for you to feel that you are no longer on the verge of orgasm. You need not, and should not, wait so long that your arousal disappears. Just pause long enough for you to feel "safe"—that you won't come as soon as you begin stimulating yourself again. Your erection may or may not subside during this pause.

When you feel that your level of arousal has dropped to where you are no longer on the verge of coming, write down the time on the Record, next to the words Stimulation 2 Start. For example:

Session 1

Stimulation 1	Start: 7:35
Pause 1	Stop: 7:45
Stimulation 2	Start: *7:46*

Now begin to stimulate yourself actively for a second time. During this second self-stimulation period, you will do the same as during the first one: get yourself aroused to a point close to orgasm and then stop stimulating yourself. If you do go over the line, and come, don't get upset. You are testing your limits here, so to speak, and you should expect to cross those limits every so often. It is better for the purposes of this program, moreover, that you sometimes go too far than not far enough. So, when you feel that you are close to climax again, *stop* actively stimulating yourself, but do not let go of your penis. Stop any looking or thinking that is getting you turned on, as well as your stroking. Look at your watch and jot down the time on your Record, beside the word Stop for Stimulation 2. For example:

Session 1

| Stimulation 1 | Start: 7:35 |
| Pause 1 | Stop: 7:45 |

| Stimulation 2 | Start: 7:46 |
| | Stop: 7:51 |

Again, stimulation period 2 is to be followed by a pause. Stop your self-stimulation just long enough for you to feel that you are no longer on the verge of orgasm—to a point where you feel it would be "safe" to touch yourself again without coming immediately. When you sense that you have reached this point, write down the time again in the Record, next to Stimulation 3 Start. For example:

Session 1

| Stimulation 1 | Start: 7:35 |
| Pause 1 | Stop: 7:45 |

| Stimulation 2 | Start: 7:46 |
| Pause 2 | Stop: 7:51 |

Stimulation 3	Start: 7:53

Repeat the same routine. This means getting yourself highly aroused to a point just short of orgasm, and then pausing. The amount of time it takes you to reach this peak level of arousal for the third time is liable to be shorter than it was during stimulation periods 1 and 2. It may also be more difficult for you to pause in time to avoid coming. This is to be expected, especially during the early phases of the program, and it is nothing to be overly concerned about. As we said, it is important that you try to get close to the point of orgasm; therefore, it is better for purposes of learning if you stop too late, as opposed to stopping too soon. Also, it is important that you stop stroking yourself, but not let go of your penis, and that you resume active stimulation as soon as you feel it is safe to do so. Therefore, restarting stimulation too soon is better than restarting it too late.

When you feel that you are once again close to orgasm (that is, for the third time), pause. Again, make a note of the time in your Record. For example:

Session 1

Stimulation 1	Start: 7:35
Pause 1	Stop: 7:45

Stimulation 2	Start: 7:46
Pause 2	Stop: 7:51

Stimulation 3	Start: 7:53
	Stop: 7:55

You are now ready for the third and final pause. When you feel that your arousal has subsided to a level where you are no longer on the verge of coming, make a quick note of the time on your Record, beside the heading Stimulation 4 Start. For example:

Session 1

Stimulation 1	Start: 7:35
Pause 1	Stop: 7:45
Stimulation 2	Start: 7:46
Pause 2	Stop: 7:51
Stimulation 3	Start: 7:53
Pause 3	Stop: 7:55
Stimulation 4	Start: *7:59*

Finish the fourth and final stimulation period by bringing yourself to orgasm. Make a note of the time, as in the example below, and then lie back and relax.

Session 1

Stimulation 1	Start: 7:35
Pause 1	Stop: 7:45
Stimulation 2	Start: 7:46
Pause 2	Stop: 7:51
Stimulation 3	Start: 7:53
Pause 3	Stop: 7:55
Stimulation 4	Start: 7:59
	Stop: *8:00*

You have now finished Session 1.

After you have had a chance to relax for a while, go through your Stimulation and Pause Record and compute the times, in minutes, for stimulation periods 1, 2, 3, and 4, and for pauses

1, 2, and 3. Use the times you wrote down for this purpose. For example:

Session 1

Stimulation 1	Start: 7:35 Stop: 7:45	10 Minutes
Pause 1		1 Minute
Stimulation 2	Start: 7:46 Stop: 7:51	5 Minutes
Pause 2		2 Minutes
Stimulation 3	Start: 7:53 Stop: 7:55	2 Minutes
Pause 3		4 Minutes
Stimulation 4	Start: 7:59 Stop: 8:00	1 Minute
Total Time		25 Minutes

This record shows that it took ten minutes for the man in this example to stimulate himself to the verge of orgasm the first time (Stimulation 1). It took one minute for his level of arousal to subside, after he stopped stimulating himself, to a point where he felt that he could resume stimulation without coming immediately (Pause 1). It took five minutes of self-stimulation to reach the verge of orgasm a second time (Stimulation 2), and two minutes of pausing for the arousal to subside to a safe level again (Pause 2). To get to the verge of orgasm a third time took only two minutes of active stimulation (Stimulation 3), and it took four minutes for this peak level to subside to a safer level (Pause 3). It took one minute to reach orgasm after the third and final pause (Stimulation 4). Altogether the man in this example was able, by using the pause technique, to go for twenty-five minutes (Total Time) before reaching orgasm.

Following this procedure may seem like a lot of work to you, and in fact it is, at least in the beginning. Having to look at a clock several times and write down the times on the Record can be an unwelcome interference at first. Also, the procedure may make you self-conscious and distract you from sexually exciting stimulation. For these reasons it may take longer to get yourself initially turned on during each session (Stimulation 1). As much of an inconvenience as it may be, however, the pause technique has been found effective in training men to delay orgasm. In addition, keeping a written record is useful in that it provides some concrete evidence of progress.

To complete Step 1, you should have *at least three* sessions like the one described above. If you have more than three (which is even better), keep a record of them so that you can continue to compute times and observe your progress. During each session, pause three times, if you can, before going on to orgasm. You can do these sessions on consecutive days if you like, but one every other day is recommended.

When you have had a chance to do several self-stimulation sessions, take a few minutes to study your records. Note first the *total time* of each session. If you were able to delay orgasm for this long during intercourse, would you be satisfied? Were you able to do three pauses each time, or did you have one or more "accidents": times when you could not pause, and came before Stimulation 4? What do you think was responsible for this: not paying attention to your level of arousal, stimulating yourself too intensely, or not pausing long enough before restarting stimulation?

Look now at the duration (length) of your stimulation periods and your pauses. Usually, at the beginning of a program like this one, men find that their stimulation periods get *shorter,* while their pauses get *longer.* It takes, in other words, less and less time to get to the verge of orgasm, and more and more time for your level of arousal to subside to where it is safe to resume

STIMULATION AND PAUSE RECORD: STEP 1

	Session 1		Session 2		Session 3
Stimulation 1	Start: Stop:	⌒ ___ Minutes ___ Minutes	Start: Stop:	⌒ ___ Minutes ___ Minutes	Start: Stop:	⌒ ___ Minutes ___ Minutes
Pause 1					
Stimulation 2	Start: Stop:	⌒ ___ Minutes ___ Minutes	Start: Stop:	⌒ ___ Minutes ___ Minutes	Start: Stop:	⌒ ___ Minutes ___ Minutes
Pause 2					
Stimulation 3	Start: Stop:	⌒ ___ Minutes	Start: Stop:	⌒ ___ Minutes	Start: Stop:	⌒ ___ Minutes
Stimulation 4	Start: Stop:	⌒ ___ Minutes	Start: Stop:	⌒ ___ Minutes	Start: Stop:	⌒ ___ Minutes
Total Time		___ Minutes		___ Minutes		___ Minutes

stimulation. After a few sessions, however, a trend usually appears in which the duration of your pauses will tend to decrease, while your stimulation periods will become longer. This will be a reflection of improved awareness of your level of sexual arousal, which in turn leads to better "control" of that arousal. With sufficient practice you may be able to pause four, five, six, or more times before going on to orgasm. This, too, would reflect your improving awareness and control.

If you do not feel that you have developed good control by doing the minimum of three self-stimulation sessions, or if you have more than one "accident," have a few more sessions before moving on to Step 2. In addition, even as you progress through this program, you should continue to practice the pause technique, with at least one pause, each time you masturbate. This is important practice that will contribute in the long run to your ability to delay orgasm during sexual encounters.

Step 2

For Step 2 of the program you will need a partner. If you are married, living with someone, or are single but have a steady sexual partner, your program partner should be that woman. Hopefully, she will have read this material, and together you will have decided that it is in your mutual interest to help you learn to delay orgasm.

Now you will need the Stimulation and Pause Record: Step 2, which follows. It is similar to the record used in Step 1. There is, however, one major difference; in the sessions for Step 2, you will be doing only two pauses.

Instead of stimulating yourself as in Step 1, in Step 2 your partner should be the one to stimulate you. And she should do this in a specific way—while you are lying on your back, using only her hands. You should spread your legs slightly apart.

The sessions you and your partner should have will be similar to the ones you did in Step 1. You will be using the same pause procedure. As before, during each stimulation period, you should get sexually aroused, by having your penis stroked by your partner, to a level that feels close to orgasm. Then you are to pause. You will probably need to tell your partner how to stroke you, and you will also need to give her a clear signal when you want her to stop stimulating you.

When you pause, your partner should stop stroking you, but she should not let go of your penis. At the same time you should stop fantasizing, watching the action, or doing anything else that contributes to your sexual arousal.

You might begin these sessions with a sensual massage, as described in chapter 6. Beginning this way, rather than with genital stimulation, is pleasant and relaxing for both partners. Men who are concerned about their sexual performance tend to be very up-tight in bed. This can not only be distracting, but may actually add to a tendency to reach orgasm quickly. Also, couples sometimes report that it feels uncomfortably mechanical to just hop into bed and begin the pause technique. Devoting time to becoming relaxed and enjoying one another before starting the pause procedure is worthwhile.

Again, you will be keeping track of time during your sessions, so have a clock or watch handy. However, let your partner keep the record now. The example in Step 1 will show her how to do this. After you have finished each session, compute the times for stimulations and pauses, and take a look at the results. This is a good way for you to watch your own progress.

It is more likely that you will have one or more "accidents"—times when you cannot pause quickly enough, and you will have an orgasm—during Step 2 than during Step 1. This is partly because being stroked by a partner is usually more arousing than stroking yourself, and partly because you will need to develop some effective communication to be able to pause in time.

You and your partner should work on Step 2 until you are able to have *at least three* complete sessions; that is, sessions in which you pause twice before being stimulated to orgasm by your partner. After you reach orgasm you can, of course, pleasure your partner and stimulate her to orgasm in any way you would like. If you jump ahead to Step 3 before you have at least three successful sessions on this step, you are not likely to do well on it. It may take you more than three tries before you can reach the goals of Step 2 and be in a position to move ahead. Give yourself as much time as you need.

When you have finished a number of sessions together, look at the length of the stimulation and pause periods as they appear on your record. First, look at the *totals* for the sessions. If these totals are lower than the ones for the Step 1 sessions, this, too, will be because being stimulated by your partner is more exciting for you than stimulating yourself. You should, however, note a trend toward longer totals for the later sessions. Similarly, as compared to your sessions during Step 1, chances are that the sessions with your partner have shorter stimulation periods and longer pauses. That is to be expected, again for the reason that being stimulated by your partner is often more exciting. With practice, the same trends should appear as during Step 1. You will probably notice that your pauses tend to get shorter (it will take less time for your level of arousal to subside to a "safe" point), while the length of your stimulation periods should increase.

Step 3

The goals of this step are for you to be able to penetrate your partner without immediately reaching orgasm, and then to pause twice, again using manual stimulation by your partner, before reaching orgasm.

> *Begin your sessions with a sensual massage. When you both feel ready to move on, lie down on your back, with your legs spread apart somewhat. Let your partner begin to stroke your penis, but not so that you get to a point of high arousal. Rather, she should stimulate you only to erection. Then she should straddle you, or sit on top of you. If you still have an erection then, insert your penis, with your partner's help, into her vagina. Your legs should still be spread apart at this point. If you lose your erection*

STIMULATION AND PAUSE RECORD: STEP 2

		Session 1		Session 2		Session 3
Stimulation 1	Start: Stop:	}____ Minutes ____ Minutes	Start: Stop:	}____ Minutes ____ Minutes	Start: Stop:	}____ Minutes ____ Minutes
Pause 1						
Stimulation 2	Start: Stop:	}____ Minutes ____ Minutes	Start: Stop:	}____ Minutes ____ Minutes	Start: Stop:	}____ Minutes ____ Minutes
Pause 2						
Stimulation 3	Start: Stop:	}____ Minutes ____ Minutes	Start: Stop:	}____ Minutes ____ Minutes	Start: Stop:	}____ Minutes ____ Minutes
Total Time		____ Minutes		____ Minutes		____ Minutes

while your partner moves around to straddle you, let her stroke you again until you are erect, and then penetrate her.

Once you are inside your partner, you should both be still. Try not to move very much. Don't worry if you lose your erection. Your goal is simply to be able to penetrate and stay inside of your partner for a while without coming. Moving around will stimulate your penis even more than being still, which is the reason to avoid it. The difficulty with this step is that penetration itself tends to be a highly arousing event, both physically and psychologically; therefore, being still together after you penetrate is, in effect, a pause.

If you are able to penetrate your partner without coming, and you can be still together for a minute without you reaching orgasm, slowly close your legs. This may increase your level of arousal, and if you feel yourself getting close to orgasm, spread your legs again, then try closing them once more when your arousal subsides.

It may happen that you come immediately after penetrating your partner, or even as you are penetrating her. If so, don't get upset. If the same thing happens the second time you try Step 3, go back to Step 2 and do some additional sessions, and then return to this step.

If you continue to come either right after or while you are penetrating your partner, even after repeating Step 2, there are several things you can do. The first is to consider whether you may be letting your partner get you too highly aroused before attempting penetration. You can try penetrating her earlier; you may even try penetrating before you have a full erection. Second, you can try wearing a condom, since this tends to reduce the amount of stimulation to the glans of your penis. Third, you can ask your partner to use some sort of vaginal lubricant, some men find lubricants decrease arousal. This should be a water-soluble gel, available in drugstores. Finally, you can try spreading your legs apart more and also bending them at the knees, since this position is usually less arousing for men than lying with your legs closer together and straight.

> *Once you have been able to penetrate your partner and be still together for a minute or so without reaching orgasm, remove your penis. Do **not** pump together or otherwise attempt to reach orgasm while you are in her.*
>
> *When you are out of your partner, ask her to stimulate you with her hands until you sense that you are close to orgasm, as she did in Step 2, and then pause until your arousal subsides to a safe level. Ask your partner to begin stimulating you again, then pause a second time. The third time she stimulates you, let her continue until you reach orgasm. Afterward you can change places and stimulate her to orgasm in any ways that the two of you choose.*

When you and your partner have been able to complete the above *twice consecutively,* you may move on to Step 4. Do not proceed to the next step until you can insert your penis into your partner's vagina, with her on top, and not reach orgasm, and then be manually stimulated to a peak of arousal twice before you reach orgasm. It may take some time before you are able to complete a session like this twice in a row, but that is what you should be able to do before you move to Step 4.

Step 4

By now you should be experiencing a greater sense of control over your sexual arousal. If you often came before, during, or right after penetration, you have already accomplished a great deal by making it through Step 3 successfully.

In Step 4, your goal is to be able to use the pause technique with your penis inside of your partner's vagina.

> *Begin your sessions with a sensual massage. When you and your partner feel ready, begin touching to get each other turned on, but not to a point close to orgasm (at least not for you). When you are both feeling turned on and when you have an erection, ask your partner to straddle you, and penetrate her in that position. Then be still for a moment.*

If you don't feel that you are on the verge of orgasm, spread your legs slightly and bend them at the knee. Then, while you lie still, let your partner begin to move. Starting with very slow pumping movements, let her stimulate your penis in this way until you feel your level of arousal rise. If this does not happen, ask your partner to move a little faster, until you feel yourself getting more aroused. If you still don't sense yourself getting very excited, try straightening out your legs and/or closing them.

Let your partner continue to pump against your penis until your arousal gets to the point, which is probably familar to you by now, where you sense that orgasm is close. Then tell her to stop pumping. She should try to do this immediately and then sit still on top of you while your arousal subsides. If need be, you can spread your legs and bend them as additional ways of reducing your arousal. Also, stop any fantasies or other sexually exciting thoughts. Pause in this manner until your arousal subsides to a level where you feel that your partner can begin stimulating you by pumping again.

Let your partner move against you until you reach the verge of orgasm a second time, then pause again as described above. When your arousal has subsided to a safe level again, ask your partner to begin moving once more. This time she may continue to move, and you may, too, until you reach orgasm. Then it will be your turn to pleasure her.

As you can see, what you and your partner are doing in Step 4 is very similar to what you did alone in Step 1 and with her in Step 2. The general idea is that you will monitor your own level of arousal and learn to detect when you are close to orgasm. Hopefully you can arrange, by being careful enough, for your arousal to build slowly, so that you will have time to pause when you sense that you are close to coming. When you pause, you delay orgasm.

You and your partner should continue to work on Step 4 until you are able to have *at least three* of these sessions, each of which includes two pauses prior to orgasm. Initially you will probably find that your arousal follows a familiar pattern, with your stimulation periods being shorter and shorter and your pauses longer and longer. As you have more sessions together, familiar trends should appear: your stimulation periods (when your partner is pumping against you) will increase, while your pauses get shorter. It can take some time for this sort of control to develop, and there may be occasional "accidents," but it will be well worth your while to stick with it until you sense that these changes are taking place.

Step 5

By following this step-by-step procedure, you have learned to delay orgasm through the use of the pause technique. This requires both patience and cooperation between you and your partner. Underlying all must be a belief on both your parts that you each stand to gain something from the effort put into the program.

If you have progressed according to instructions and not jumped ahead, you should now be able to delay orgasm when you and your partner have intercourse in the woman-on-top position. Also, up to this point your partner has been the one to do the moving, while you lie back and monitor your level of arousal so that you can tell her when to pause. Now you should experiment with changing positions and with you doing some of the moving. Both of these changes are likely to increase your overall level of arousal; therefore, pausing in time may once again be difficult to do at first. Don't let this discourage you.

> *Start your lovemaking sessions in whatever way you like. Get each other turned on, but your partner should still not get you so aroused that you are close to coming before you attempt penetration. If necessary, use the pause technique during foreplay to control your level of arousal.*
>
> *When you have an erection, let your partner lie on her back while you penetrate her from the man-on-top position. Do this with your legs slightly spread. If you do not come immediately, but are able to penetrate, lie on top of your partner and spread your*

legs wider. Also, bend them slightly at the knees. This should serve to reduce your level of arousal. Lie still in this position for a minute and don't worry if your erection subsides a little.

If you come during, or right after, penetration, try again later or the next day. If this happens persistently, return to Step 4 and work on developing your control more in the woman-on-top position, and then return to Step 5.

After lying still for a minute or so, begin moving very slowly. Ask your partner to lie still while you thrust, slowly, with your legs slightly spread. Thrust until you sense that you are on the verge of orgasm, then pause by lying still. When your arousal has subsided to a safe level, begin slow thrusting again. If you can, pause a second time. Then thrust at a pace that is comfortable to you until you reach orgasm, and afterwards lie still again. Note the position of your legs and the angle at which you were thrusting; this will tell you what is the most sexually arousing intercourse position for you, at least when you are on top of your partner.

Because she is being asked to lie still and focus on you, your partner may not be able to reach orgasm during these sessions. You may, of course, pleasure her as much as you and she like after you come.

After you penetrate your partner from the man-on-top position, you may find that your level of arousal jumps quickly to a peak, with little or no thrusting, and that it is difficult for you to pause in time. This is most likely to happen the first couple of times you try penetrating from this position. If a pattern of quick orgasm persists, however, you can experiment with some of the things mentioned earlier. For instance, you can return to Step 4 for a while and try to develop more control. But try this first. If the pattern persists, experiment with any or all of the following: wearing a condom, asking your partner to use a water-soluble vaginal lubricant, penetrating earlier, for instance, when you are only partially erect, and finally, pausing sooner. Each of these things should tend to reduce your level of arousal at the time of penetration.

Once you are inside of your partner and thrusting, it may be possible for you to adjust your level of arousal, and also the rate at which your arousal builds, by varying *your position.* Men usually find that some intercourse positions are more arousing than others. *That is why you should make a mental note of your position when you finally thrust to orgasm during the sessions in this step. The position you choose—the position of your legs and the angle of thrusting—will be one that is most arousing for you. Knowing this, you can then adjust your arousal by moving* away from *this very arousing position. For example, if you notice that you thrust to orgasm with your legs tightly closed and with your penis moving almost straight up and down, you will probably find that your arousal builds more slowly when you thrust with your legs slightly apart and when your penis thrusts at a different angle. Experiment with this, even if you are able to pause twice before reaching orgasm; it will give you yet another way of controlling your arousal, thus delaying orgasm.*

It will probably take some time to learn to pause and delay orgasm when you are in the missionary, or man-on-top, position, and when you are doing the moving. You may need to work on learning to adjust your body position and on pausing earlier than you have been accustomed to. The length of your stimulation periods may be very short at first, but with practice they should gradually lengthen. Similarly, your pauses may be long at first, that is, it may take some time for your arousal to subside to a level where it would be safe to start thrusting again without coming immediately. In time, however, your pauses should become briefer.

In the end, the degree to which you will be able to delay orgasm depends on how much practice you put into it. In general, the more often you repeat the pause procedure, and the more pauses you do each time, the better you will get at it and the longer you will be able to delay. Progress in this direction, however, is usually slow but steady, so don't expect too much too soon. Also, you may expect to experience some "accidents" or even temporary setbacks—periods when your control seems poorer than it has been. This will simply reflect the fact that your sexual response is not something constant, but rather something that fluctuates. Sometimes (and occasionally for periods of time) you may be more highly aroused (or arousable) than usual; it is during these times that you are likely to experience poorer control. In addition, the length of time between orgasms and sexual encounters is a factor to be considered. If you have not had an orgasm in several days, or if you have not been in bed with a woman for a while, you will be prone to coming more quickly during your next sexual encounter.

When you and your partner have worked on Step 5 for a while, and you feel that you have developed some ability to control your arousal and delay orgasm, you may want to turn your attention to the broader issue of sexual fulfillment within your relationship. Many of the earlier exercises in this book are designed to help you move beyond the level of being sexually "functional" toward a greater sense of sexual fulfillment. You should read this material and experiment with the exercises.

SUMMARY

Information gathered by sex researchers shows that a number of men have a natural tendency to reach orgasm fairly quickly, especially during intercourse. Although this does not seem to represent an abnormal condition, many men whose natural response is to reach orgasm quickly are interested in learning to delay orgasm, partly for their own satisfaction and partly to please their partners. The goal of this chapter is to provide a program for accomplishing this, using a step-by-step approach. The core of the training program involves learning a pause technique, in which you control your arousal by first learning to monitor it as it rises slowly. Essentially, you practice letting your arousal build and then letting it subside by cutting off sources of erotic stimulation. This is not necessarily an easy skill to develop, and it requires motivation, patience, and persistence.

In the early stages of the program, you work by yourself, but further progress requires the willing cooperation of an interested partner. The later exercises are designed to guide you as a couple toward reaching a common goal, one you both desire. This is another illustration of the fact that sexual fulfillment is not something we can effectively pursue as isolated individuals, but rather is something best accomplished in the context of a relationship.

Sometimes just learning to delay orgasm longer than you have been able to in the past is the sole sexual goal that a man, or a couple, may have. More often, however, it is only part of what he or they would like to achieve in the way of sexual satisfaction. The earlier chapters of this book explore the broader goal of sexual fulfillment. Once you have accomplished your initial goal of learning to delay orgasm, you should explore these further possibilities for sexual fulfillment.

11 learning to accelerate orgasm

Just as there are men whose natural tendency is to reach orgasm quickly, and without a great deal of stimulation, so there are individuals whose normal pattern is to reach orgasm more slowly and only after a great deal of stimulation. In addition, men experience variations in their sexual responsiveness, so that sometimes they may reach orgasm more quickly, and after less stimulation, than at other times. Such variations are normal, and probably have to do with a number of physical factors (health, diet, and fatigue) as well as psychological factors (your mood, the particular circumstances under which sex occurs, the quality of your relationship at the time, and so on). Occasional experiences with reaching orgasm either more quickly or more slowly than you would like are therefore not "sexual dysfunctions" and should not be a cause for concern.

Even though there are normally variations in men's sexual responsiveness, we are usually aware of how much stimulation, on the average, it takes for us to reach orgasm. We know, for example, how long and how much pressure is needed in stroking our penises to orgasm. Similarly, we are accustomed to reaching orgasm, with a particular partner, after having intercourse for a certain amount of time. To some men this average amount of time it takes to reach orgasm (especially through intercourse) seems too short. But for others, reaching the point of orgasm seems to take too long, and so they are interested in learning to accelerate the process. That is what this chapter is about.

SETTING GOALS

There are limits on the extent to which people can change their natural sexual response pattern. There are limits, in other words, on how much a man can learn to delay orgasm, and there are limits as well on how much his orgasm can be accelerated. It is important to realize this and to set your goals accordingly. Don't expect yourself to be able to control your sexual responsiveness totally. Expect, rather, to be able to modify your responsiveness a bit in one direction or another. Specifically, this chapter will discuss techniques which you can use to facilitate your sexual arousal, and others which can help reduce or eliminate factors which interfere with your arousal. Together, these techniques can teach you how to reach orgasm somewhat more quickly than you have in the past. In the course of your sex life, however, you can expect to continue to experience variations, so that there will always be times when you reach orgasm more slowly than others.

PLAN OF THE PROGRAM

Men who feel that it takes too long and/or too much stimulation for them to reach orgasm, often feel frustrated and angry or depressed. They feel that sex, rather than being fun, has become too much like work for them (and maybe for their partners, too); as a result they may lose interest in it. Sometimes they fear that their partners will lose interest in them, and leave them for a man who has less "trouble" coming. Understandably, this kind of fear can put a great strain on a relationship. Not infrequently, concern over difficulty in reaching orgasm turns into self-consciousness and performance anxiety, which leads in turn to erection problems. If this is true for you, so that you have gotten to the point where you've developed an erection problem, you need to work on that before learning to accelerate orgasm. Chapters 8 and 9 are devoted to dealing with erection problems, and you should turn to them now.

Essentially, learning to accelerate orgasm requires work in three separate areas. The first of these concerns your overall physical condition. You need to appreciate the connection between physical health and sexual responsiveness, and perhaps to do something in the interests of both. The second area involves working to eliminate or minimize interferences, psychological factors that get in the way of your ability to get sexually aroused. This is the issue of complications, which has been discussed before (chapter 8). It would be helpful if you were to review that material now. The third thing you need to be able to do in order to accelerate orgasm is to be able to increase your level of sexual arousal. This involves learning to utilize different channels of arousal, a topic which was discussed in the previous chapter. In this case you need to discover ways of maximizing the sources of sexual arousal available to you.

Getting in Shape

People often neglect the fact that sex, aside from its emotional significance, is a physical act. Like any physical act you engage in, your sexual performance will be affected by your overall physical condition. If you neglect your body, in other words, your sexual performance will suffer. This is a common-sense notion, yet many people who complain of sexual difficulties seem to ignore it. On the one hand they may understand perfectly well that a person may not perform well or have fun jogging or playing tennis if he or she is out of shape. On the other hand, they often fail to apply this same sort of thinking toward sex. Yet physical fitness certainly does matter. Your sexual performance, as well as the pleasure you derive from your sex life, will be influenced significantly by your state of health and physical condition.

Many of the men I've worked with who complain of difficulties in reaching orgasm have not been in particularly good physical condition for their age. It is not that they are ill, but they are not physically fit. They may be overweight, drink and/or smoke too much, and get little or no regular exercise. Like many people, they limit sex to late at night when they are already tired. Under such circumstances it is little wonder that they experience difficulties getting or staying aroused, or in getting sufficiently aroused to experience orgasm.

As a first step in changing your sexual responsiveness so that you can accelerate orgasm, you need to seriously reevaluate your physical fitness. Are you in decent condition or not? If not, then don't expect your sexual performance to be as good as it might be, or as good as it was when you were more fit.

If you have let yourself go, physically speaking, you should consider doing something about it for the sake of your health in general and your sex life in particular. However, you need to go about doing this intelligently. If you are out of shape, diving into a pool and swimming until you are exhausted, or jogging until you collapse, is not the way to improve things. It took time for you to get out of shape, and it will take time for you to get into shape. There are several books on exercise and conditioning; I suggest you get one and read it. Do this *before* starting on a fitness program. If you have any physical ailments, you should also consult with your physician before you begin. Select a program that is appropriate for your age and overall health, and then follow it. Don't expect immediate results, sexually or otherwise. In the long run, however, your efforts should prove very worthwhile.

Minimizing Complications

I have used the term *complications* to refer to various psychological factors that can interfere with sexual arousal. For men whose difficulty has to do with not reaching orgasm, or reaching orgasm very slowly, the most common complication is self-conscious worry, or performance anxiety. These men often get into a vicious cycle in which they approach sex anxiously. As I've said before, lying in a bed worrying about your sexual performance is not a sexually exciting activity. You cannot expect yourself to feel sexually aroused if you spend your time worrying about whether or not you'll come, any more than you would get excited if you were to lie there worrying about your unpaid bills. You need to break out of this cycle, in which worrying about your sexual performance undermines that performance, if you are to have any chance of improving your situation.

The greatest source of frustration that men in this situation experience stems from the fact that they seem to have their minds set on reaching orgasm only through intercourse. As pleasant as this experience is, if you make it the only acceptable way of reaching orgasm, you are placing frustrating limits on yourself. As much as men might enjoy reaching orgasm through intercourse, I would suggest that there are different ways of reaching orgasm that can be equally intense and pleasant experiences. Being able to reach orgasm, for instance, by using a vibrator, through oral sex, or by stimulating yourself in your partner's presence, can be a very intimate and exciting experience. Developing a sexual relationship that is open to such experiences, however, depends on the motivation of two people. If you are not open to the possibility that these forms of sex can be exciting, intense, fulfilling, and fun, you are limiting the number of ways through which you and your partner can achieve sexual intimacy. Equally important, this attitude—that orgasm must occur through intercourse or not at all—will make it more difficult for you to break out of your self-defeating cycle of worry. The exercises in chapter 3 should help in this regard. Through developing your sexual repertoire you will not only be expanding your sources of pleasure; you will also be working toward minimizing the complications caused by a narrow view of sexuality.

A second common complication experienced by men who are having difficulty reaching orgasm is that they are usually tense, right from the beginning, during their sexual encounters. During intercourse they become especially tense, both mentally and physically. Sometimes they are so physically tense that they experience muscle cramps in their arms or legs. This is a sign that they are working too hard at trying to overcome worry. They are trying to push themselves, by brute force, to the point of orgasm. If they succeed, it is usually exhausting, and less than satisfying in the long run. To break out of a tendency to be so tense during sex that it interferes with your sexual arousal, you need to learn to apply a specific relaxation technique (see chapter 5). It will take you a little time to learn, but it will be worth the effort.

In addition to worrying about his sexual performance and trying to force his arousal, a man's sexual excitement, and therefore his chances of reaching orgasm, can be undermined by a number of other complicating factors. One such factor is fear, for example, the fear of getting a partner pregnant. This fear may not be strong enough to interfere with his getting or keeping an erection, but it may be intense enough to inhibit a man's ability to reach orgasm. Most often the strength of this fear increases as his level of excitement builds. Therefore his fear will be greatest when he is closest to orgasm. Naturally, this will undermine his arousal, and the man will experience difficulty in reaching climax.

Several psychological factors which can inhibit sexual arousal, like fear of pregnancy, are discussed in chapter 8, along with strategies for dealing with these sorts of complications. It is important that you review this material. Consider which, if any, of these factors may be interfering with your ability to get maximally aroused, and work at minimizing them.

Maximizing Arousal

In chapter 10 a strategy for manipulating your level of arousal by experimenting with different channels of stimulation was outlined. In that chapter the sexual goal was to help men learn to delay orgasm by decreasing their level of arousal as they neared the point of climax. The same techniques described there, if used in reverse, can help men who want to learn the opposite, that is, to accelerate orgasm. Your goal is to *maximize* the number of sources of arousal available to you. The more such sources you can use, and the less your attention drifts away from them, the higher your level of sexual excitement will be. Several specific techniques that can be used toward this end (some of which are described in chapter 10) include:

> *Extended Foreplay* Make your foreplay longer and more intense, so that your level of arousal is already high when you have intercourse. Experiment with using a vibrator, on each other or on yourself. This can be a very pleasurable and intense form of stimulation. There are times when you may need such intense stimulation in order to reach orgasm. This does not mean that you are abnormal, only that your natural pattern is inclined toward a little more stimulation.
>
> *Touching During Intercourse* Ask your partner to stroke or squeeze your penis with her fingers while you have intercourse. She may be able to do this fairly easily if you have intercourse in the woman-on-top position, in a side-by-side position, or in a scissors position in which you lie side by side with your bodies forming an "X". Your partner may even be able to use a vibrator to stimulate you in the scissors position.
>
> *Watching or Fantasizing* Men frequently report that watching

their partner while she touches them or watching themselves make love, for example, in a mirror, adds to their sexual excitement. Similarly, imagining a sexually exciting scene usually adds to a man's arousal (see the discussion on fantasies in chapter 4). You might consider experimenting with either of these techniques.

Shifting Positions Men usually find that certain intercourse positions are more sexually stimulating for them than others. Of course, the sorts of positions that are available to you depends on both you and your partner. Experiment with a variety of positions to find those that are most exciting to both of you. Two specific things that the man should try varying are the position of his legs (open or closed) and the angle of penetration of his penis in his partner's vagina.

Sensory Focus Each one of our senses has erotic potential. The feelings in your body when you are touched, the way your partner's body looks and feels, the way she moves, the sounds she makes, and so on can all be sexually exciting. Experiment with shifting your attention from one sensory channel to another. See if you find some things particularly exciting.

Communication Men often say that being talked to, as well as talking to their partner during lovemaking, is a turn-on. Experiment with telling your partner how much she turns you on, and what it is specifically about her body that appeals to you. Tell her what you like doing to her, and how it feels as you are doing it. If you like the feeling of having your penis inside of her, say so. If you like kissing her breasts, tell her that. See if letting yourself express feelings adds to your arousal.

Experimenting with and developing different channels of sexual arousal will be useful only if you are able to use them fairly consistently during lovemaking. Therefore, you need to work in two areas: minimize distractions and increase sources of arousal. Your progress in these areas will most likely be slow but steady; be persistent and patient.

SUMMARY

This chapter has been devoted to the task of trying to accelerate orgasm. Men who feel that they have trouble reaching orgasm need first of all to set realistic goals for themselves in terms of how much they may be able to change. To some extent their need for prolonged and/or intense stimulation may be a natural pattern, just as some men's natural tendency is to reach orgasm fairly quickly.

If you would like to work on trying to accelerate orgasm, there are three areas to which you need to direct your attention. First, there is the matter of your overall physical condition. Physical fitness and sexual performance are related, so if you are not physically fit, don't expect your sexual performance to be as good as it might be. Second, you need to think about possible psychological factors that may be interfering with your sexual arousal during lovemaking, the most likely of these being performance anxiety. Other complicating factors, discussed in detail in chapter 8, can also interfere with your excitement. The third area in which you may need to do some work involves learning to increase the number of ways in which you get sexually turned on. The more you are able to make use of a variety of channels of stimulation, the better your chances will be of maximizing your level of arousal and facilitating orgasm.

index

A

Abstinence, 118
Affairs, 60, 61, 67, 250
Affection, 65, 121, 142, 166, 179, 180, 196, 199, 308
Afterplay, 12, 196
Aggravation, 162
Aging:
  effect of, on sexuality, 14, 239, 240
Alcohol:
  and erection problems, 291
  and physical fitness, 339
Anal intercourse, 42
Anger, 99, 109, 111, 255, 257, 302, 337
Anxiety (Nervous tension), 12, 88, 113, 116, 130, 140, 141, 142, 143, 145, 151, 157, 158, 159, 197, 198, 199, 207, 224, 225, 231, 238, 242, 246, 267, 276, 298
  about change, 38, 85
  about sharing sexual experiences, 134, 135
  about women, 110, 191
  desensitization approach to overcoming, 277–78
  of women about "sexy" men, 112
  "one jump" approach to overcoming, 277–78
  over trying to become a superlover, 25
  reactions, 204
  reducing, 202, 215
  suppression of, 143
  symptoms of, 191, 197, 204
Appearance:
  changing one's, 115–17
  personal, 113–17
  physical, of women, 44–52, 53, 56, 59, 70, 75, 310
Arguments, 165
Arousal, sexual, 3, 13, 14, 20, 71, 72, 98, 99, 101, 102, 104, 121, 123,

Arousal, sexual (*cont.*)
125, 128, 129, 133, 141, 158, 169, 172, 207, 208, 215, 219, 224, 229, 231, 241, 243, 247, 248, 252, 257, 258, 260, 261, 263, 267, 268, 270, 272, 279, 280, 281, 284, 287, 288, 289, 291, 301, 304, 306, 315, 316, 317, 319, 321, 322, 324, 325, 326, 328, 329, 332, 333, 334, 337, 338, 340, 341
and erections, 273–76
channels of stimulation and, 310–14
controlling, 309, 310
"forcing," 242
lubrication of, 223
Manipulating Your, an exercise, 313–14
maximizing, 342–44
psychic stimulation, the main source of, 13
sabotaged by jealousy, 254
sources of, 16
Asexual:
women regarded in past as, 27, 28
Attraction, sexual, 44, 46, 49, 56, 57, 58, 59, 66, 197, 198, 199, 200, 213, 241, 257, 258, 260, 263, 299, 310
Awkwardness, 82, 85, 90, 92, 141, 199, 257

B

"Backsliding" (recurrence of erection problems), 290–97
Behavioral rehearsal, 81, 85, 90, 199
Birth control, 18, 243, 244, 294 (*see also* Contraception)
Body awareness:
building, 151–54
Developing, an exercise, 152–54
Boredom, 17, 19, 40
Breasts, 7, 45, 172, 207, 208, 212, 213, 216, 219, 228, 257, 279, 280, 281, 282, 288, 343

Breathing, 132, 144, 146, 148, 154, 156, 168, 170, 173, 207, 212, 214, 215, 217, 219, 221, 222, 283, 285, 288
Buttocks, 145, 149, 154, 171

C

Caressing, 80, 81, 88, 287, 288, 311
Caring, 300
and Playing, an exercise, 176–85
Behaviors Lists, 176–79, 181, 184
Celibacy, 241
Change:
and the sexual relationship, 39, 40, 77, 78, 85, 111, 112, 141, 175
anxiety about, 38, 85
as process, 107, 143
desire to, 38, 205
in attitudes about male sexuality, 196–97
in sexual behavior, 131
in sexual repertoire, 100
of attitude toward sex, 206
Character, 44, 70, 75
and Sexual Interest, an exercise, 52–59
defined, 52–53
schema, 53
Schema Chart, 54, 55
schema, flexibility of, 56, 57, 58
schema, rigidity of, 57, 58
Climax (*see* Orgasm)
Clitoris, 28, 29, 229
stimulation of, 28–30, 230
Commitment, 61, 247, 296, 304
Communication, 64 (*see also* Sexual communication)
improving, 40
lack of, in the family, 108
of sexual preferences, 91
Conditioned relaxation response, 151, 155, 276
Condoms, 244, 328, 332
Conflicts, 33, 164, 165, 181, 188, 255, 256, 266

Contraception, 243, 294 (*see also* Birth control)
Crises:
 effect on sexual relationship of, 66–68, 294
 job, 66–67, 259
 marital, 255
Cursing, 113

D

Depression, 17, 233, 291, 337
Desensitization, 206, 215–16, 232
 approach to overcoming anxiety, 277, 278
 procedure, 209, 215, 224, 255, 272, 277, 278–90, 296, 297, 301, 302, 303
 understanding, 276–78
Diaphragm, 244
Disappointment, 17, 40, 42, 240, 248
Disclosure:
 of one's sexual history, 199–204
 of past sexual problems, 300
Disgust, 99, 191, 204, 205, 207, 257
Dissatisfaction (with sex), 1, 18, 23, 138
Distractions during lovemaking, 167, 173, 188, 258–61, 268, 270, 275, 285, 297, 315, 322, 325, 343
Divorce, 252, 253, 293, 295
Dobrin, Arthur, 36, 106, 305

E

Ejaculation, 23, 118, 133, 196, 239
 "premature" or quick, 18, 34, 194, 195, 252, 306–35, 336
Embarrassment, 89, 92, 109, 113, 122, 131, 199, 201, 202, 203, 233, 235, 245, 262, 266, 298
Erection, 14, 19, 203
 difficulties, 1, 6, 7, 12, 13, 17, 18, 32, 33, 84, 118, 193, 194, 195, 196, 204, 341
 difficulties, fear of, 139, 263, 273
 difficulties, pinpointing, 236–40
 Dysfunction Questionnaire, 236–37
 Getting, Losing and Regaining, an exercise, 273–76
 problems, assessing, 235–40
 problems, dealing with, 269–305
 problems, understanding, 233–67
 problems and sexual desire, 240–42, 248
 problems and single men, 297–304
 problems and the desensitization procedure, 278–90
 sexual arousal and, 273–76
Erogenous zones, 14, 28, 71, 282, 311, 314
Erotic potential:
 of men's bodies, 14, 21, 40, 70, 75, 76 (*see also* Sensuality, Men's)
Exclusivity, sexual, 59, 60, 61, 64, 65, 67, 68, 69, 124, 296
Exercises:
 Caring and Playing, 176–85
 Character and Sexual Interest, 52–59
 Developing Sexual Fantasy, 125–28
 Exploring Bodies, 224–31
 Exploring Yourself, 72–75
 Fears About Communicating, 81–85
 Getting, Losing and Regaining Erections, 273–76
 Learning the Relaxation Technique, 146–51
 Learning to Communicate, 85–90
 Letting Go Alone, 129–31
 Letting Go With Your Partner, 131–33
 Letting Yourself Look, 206–9
 Manipulating Your Arousal, 313–14
 mentioned, 38, 40, 77, 78, 85, 105, 107, 112, 174, 175, 197, 209, 215, 231, 249, 265, 266, 278, 280, 299
 Physical Attributes and Sexual Interest, 44–52
 Pinpointing the Difficulty, 236–40
 Pleasuring Yourself, 120–22
 Practicing Sensual Massage, 169–74

Exercises (*cont.*)
  Preludes to Sex, 165–67
  Relationships and Sexual Interest, 59–65
  Sexual Self-Disclosure, 199–204
  Sharing and Intimacy, 185–88
  Sharing Your Sexual History, 135–38
  Specialness and Sexual Interest, 65–69
  Taking Care of Business, 162–65
  Tension Versus Relaxation, 144–45
  Understanding Your Sexual Shyness, 192–99
  Using Your Imagination, 209–16
  Your Preferred Sexual Situation, 101–5
  Your Sexual Repertoire, 93–100
Experimenting, 131, 132, 173, 175, 201, 285, 287, 342, 343
Expertise, men's sexual, 83, 84, 90

F

Fantasy, 104, 121, 122–28, 129, 132, 208, 260, 272, 274, 275, 313, 314, 317, 325, 342, 343
  Developing Sexual, an exercise, 125–28
  fear of acting out a sexual, 124
  guided, 209–24
  guilt over sexual, 205
  homosexual, 111
  sharing of sexual, 135
  technique, 209
Fatigue, 285, 291, 336
Fear(s), 41, 87, 142
  about Communicating, an exercise, 81–85
  defined, 243
  desire to overcome, 276
  intensity of, 243, 248
  of acting out a sexual fantasy, 124
  of awkwardness, 82
  of becoming a sex fiend, 26
  of communicating, 90
  of embarrassment, 298
  of erection difficulties, 139, 263, 273
  of "failing," 194, 199, 245, 293, 298, 300
  of getting caught, 295
  of involvement, 199, 246, 248, 298, 299
  of one's own sexuality, 109, 111
  of pregnancy, 18, 243, 244, 245, 247, 294, 341
  of promiscuity, 111
  of rejection, 82, 191, 192, 193, 196, 199, 201
  rooted in performance anxiety, 198
  of sex, 18, 110, 268, 299
  of sexual difficulties/dysfunction, 193, 197, 261
  of waking children during lovemaking, 104
  of women, 100, 139, 307, 308
  of women, overcoming, 190–232
  of women's bodies, 98, 257, 270
Fidelity, 60, 67
Flexibility:
  necessary for sexual fulfillment, 22, 24, 104
  of Character Schema, 56, 57, 58
  of Physical Attributes Schema, 48, 50, 51
  of sexual relationships, 291
Flirting/Flirtations, 60, 113, 160, 256
"Focusing" attention:
  on the sexually exciting, 261, 275, 285
Fondling, 3, 7, 72, 80
Foreplay, 71, 196, 203, 257, 262
  creative, 12
  extended, 342
Foreskin, 74
Frequency ratings:
  of specific sexual activities, 96, 97, 98, 99
Freud, Sigmund, 28
Frustration, 14, 16, 18, 19, 23, 26, 27–28, 35, 42, 101, 138, 159, 234, 240, 257, 262, 272, 279, 284, 302, 308, 309, 337

G

Genital focus, 14, 71, 175, 176, 189
Genital phobia, 204, 205, 215, 224, 258
Genitals, 3, 7, 72, 73, 74, 84, 98, 121, 129, 130, 145, 149, 158, 171, 172, 191, 204, 207, 213, 214, 216, 217, 221, 222, 224, 225, 226, 228, 229, 230, 231, 257, 274, 280, 281, 282, 285, 287, 288
Guilt, 89, 110, 113, 115, 116, 122, 128, 186, 193, 205, 238, 248–52, 260, 270, 275, 295, 296

H

Homosexual:
  fantasies, 111
  rape, 114
Homosexuality:
  accusation of, 257–58
  latent, 234
Hostility, 17
Hypnosis, 264

I

Ideals, sexual, 1, 26, 27
Ignorance, sexual, 28, 30, 109
Imagination, 87, 88, 200, 313, 314, 343
  Using Your, two exercises, 209–24
Immaturity:
  personal, and sexual dysfunction, 32, 33
Infidelity, 60
Inhibitions, sexual, 104, 109, 111, 112, 113, 133, 193, 232, 265
  and communication, 92
  and modesty, 115
  and self-consciousness, 114
  during the sexual encounter, 110
Instinct, 70, 75, 242
Intercourse, 19, 28, 83, 118, 203, 231, 234, 237, 244, 255, 262, 278, 279, 281, 282, 291, 295, 304, 306, 307, 322, 334, 337, 340
  anal, 42
  as achievement/accomplishment, 3, 20
  male preoccupation with, 3, 20, 71, 308
  masturbation preferred to, 119, 123
  positions, 289, 332, 333, 343
  reaching orgasm simultaneously during, 26, 27
  touching during, 342
  women who can't reach orgasm through, 29, 30
Intimacy, 22, 167, 284, 340
  patterns of, and sexual fulfillment, 174–88
  Sharing and, an exercise, 185–88
Intrauterine device (I.U.D.), 294
Involvement:
  fear of, 199, 246, 248, 298, 299

J

Jealousy, 64, 260, 270
  resentment and, 252–57
Job pressures:
  effect on sex life of, 66–67, 259

K

Kinsey sex researchers, 306
Kissing, 3, 7, 42, 72, 86, 173, 180, 197, 343

L

Lady Chatterley's Lover, 27, 30
Lawrence, D. H., 27, 31
Learning to Communicate, an exercise, 85–90
Letting Yourself be Sexual, an exercise, 108–17
Life style, 53
  celibate, 241
  self-destructive, 66
Loneliness, 12, 41, 142
Love, 31, 33, 41, 64, 142, 246, 247, 250, 254, 295

Love (*cont.*)
  communicating, 119
  simultaneous orgasm as, a sexual myth, 26–28
Lovemaking, 3, 16, 21, 108, 129, 133, 162, 163, 165, 203, 230, 273, 284, 287, 291, 292, 344
  abilities, seeking praise for, 22
  according to sexual scripts, 19, 79
  after sensual massage, 173, 174
  as mere genital pleasure, 119
  competitive, 24
  distractions during, 167, 173, 188, 258–61, 268, 270, 275, 285, 297, 315, 322, 325, 343
  fear of waking the children during, 104
  imagining, 87, 88
  in romantic, relaxed atmosphere, 188
  limited to a single pattern, 20, 22, 35, 39–40, 82
  new patterns of, 78
  skills, 15, 20, 78, 85, 91, 92, 308
  talking during, 132, 343
Lovers, 61, 62, 63, 83, 89, 90, 201, 254, 258, 264, 265, 301
Lubrication, 223, 230, 328, 332

M

Machines:
  men as sexual, 6, 11, 43, 83, 84, 174, 195, 232, 233, 242, 291
Marriage, 59, 250, 256, 260, 262, 293, 295
  counseling, 59, 65, 165, 294
  "open," 61, 62, 63, 64, 65
Masturbation, 113, 114, 118–22, 129–31, 236, 274, 275, 306
  a natural right, 119
  delaying ejaculation during, 23
  fantasizing during, 123, 126, 128, 129
  permissive attitudes toward, 249
  preferred to intercourse, 119, 123

shame over, 122, 205
  sharing experiences in, 134, 135
  stimulation for, 208
  superstitions about, 118, 122
  to orgasm, 75, 118, 122, 130
Maturity, 31, 32
  coital orgasm as, 28
Meditation, 168
"Men's" magazines, 12, 83, 116, 126, 129, 206, 207, 208, 209, 293, 313, 314, 316, 317
Mental health professionals, 31
Mirrors, 73, 101
  making love in, 343
"Modeling" sexual preferences, 91
Modesty, 53, 113, 258
  and sexual inhibition, 115
Monogamy, 59, 60, 61, 62, 63, 64
Morality, 111, 249, 251, 252
Mothers-in-law, 254–56
Myths, sexual, 26–34, 70, 80, 82, 84, 100, 194, 195, 196, 233, 240, 267

N

Nervous tension (*see* Anxiety)
Nipples, 42, 121, 172, 208, 212, 219, 228, 229, 311

O

Objectification:
  of women, 52
Openness, 186
Oral sex, 257, 340
Orgasm, 19, 22, 60, 133, 158, 175, 195, 196, 230, 275, 280, 281, 283, 284, 285, 286, 288, 289, 290, 291
  achieved by women through masturbation, 23
  clitoral, 28
  clitoral stimulation generally necessary for, 229
  coital, as "maturity," 28–30
  ending the sexual encounter upon achieving, 71

Orgasm (*cont.*)
  inability to reach, 17, 18
  internal contractions accompanying, 118
  learning to accelerate, 336–44
  learning to delay, 306–35, 342
  masturbating to, 75, 118, 122, 130
  multiple, 12
  mystical meaning of, 27
  problems, 1
  reaching, 16
  release of, 159
  second erection after, 239
  simultaneous, 30
  simultaneous, as "true love," 26–28
  vaginal, 28
  women's loss of ability to experience, 32, 33
  women who don't experience, during intercourse, 18, 29, 30

P

Passion, 31, 110, 308
Passive receiver role, 82, 84, 87
Penetration, 13, 223, 226, 230, 288, 289, 307, 310, 326, 328, 329, 332, 343
Penis, 8, 28, 71, 73, 74, 121, 122, 130, 149, 201, 204, 213, 217, 222, 230, 234, 235, 245, 246, 249, 262, 267, 270, 272, 273, 275, 279, 281, 282, 283, 285, 286, 287, 288, 292, 307, 313, 314, 317, 318, 319, 324, 325, 326, 329, 333, 337, 342, 343
  circumsized, 74
  foreskin of, 74
  glans of, 14, 28, 74, 229, 311, 312, 328
  shaft of, 74
Performance, 12, 40, 191, 202, 232, 239, 248, 251, 270, 283, 284, 289, 290, 291, 293, 295, 297, 304, 306, 307, 338, 339, 340, 341, 344
  affected by circumstances, 11
  concern with, 13, 24, 72, 276, 325
  improving, 35
  problems, 11, 31
  sex regarded as, 11, 20, 22, 24–25, 71, 84, 140, 141, 157, 158
Performance anxiety, 35, 140, 141, 157, 192, 193, 194, 195, 196, 202, 203, 204, 255, 260, 261–63, 268, 270, 278, 279, 282, 283, 285, 291, 293, 294, 295, 296, 297, 301, 303, 304, 338, 340, 344
  defined, 11
  fear rooted in, 198
  inescapable for men in our culture, 13
  minimizing, 269
  overcoming, 272
Perfume, 213
Personal:
  attraction vs. sexual attraction, 58
  fulfillment, 18, 290
  property, women as, 253, 254
  qualities, 52, 53, 54, 56, 57, 58, 59
  sensitivity, 90
Personality, 55, 56, 57, 58, 59, 187, 293, 310
Physical:
  condition, 338, 339, 344
  fitness, 339, 344
  health, 338
Physical attributes:
  and Sexual Interest, an exercise, 44–52
  of women, 44–52
  schema, 54, 55, 56, 57, 58
  Schema Chart, 46, 47
  schema, flexibility of, 48, 50, 51
  schema, rigidity of, 49, 50, 51
Platonic relationships, 194, 197
Playboy magazine, 206, 293
Pleasant Activities Lists, 181, 182–84, 185
Pleasure, 6, 18, 21, 22, 27, 28, 41, 42, 61, 70, 71, 88, 91, 92, 130, 161, 222, 242, 249, 274, 282, 339
  lovemaking as mere genital, 119

Pleasure (*cont.*)
  ratings, 94, 97, 98
Pleasuring:
  each other, 281
  self-, 23, 274–75, 314
  Yourself, an exercise, 120–22
Pornographic:
  films, 31
  pictures/stories, 123, 126
  (*see also* "Men's" magazines, Pornography)
Pornography:
  hard-core, 83, 274
  soft-core, 206, 274
  strong interest in, 111
  vs. reality, 84
Positions, intercourse, 289, 332, 333, 343
Potency, 235
Pregnancy:
  fear of, 18, 243, 244, 245, 247, 294, 341
Preludes:
  romantic, to sex, 5, 160, 162, 165, 166, 167, 189
  to Sex, an exercise, 165–67
Promiscuity, 25, 109, 111
Prostate problems, 118
Prostitution, 60, 61, 62
Prowess, sexual, 140
Psychiatric social worker, 290
Psychiatrists, 31, 290
Psychologists, 31, 290, 376
Pubic hair, 73, 208, 213, 221, 222, 228, 229
Punishment:
  external, 191, 192
  internal, 191, 192

R

Rape, 114
Recreational sex, 61, 62, 63, 87
Rejection, 82, 191, 192, 193, 196, 199, 201, 300
Relax, Learning to, 139–57

Relaxation, 180, 187, 188, 206, 212, 215, 216, 218, 219, 221, 222, 224, 226, 227, 258, 259, 276, 287, 303, 325
  planning for, 167–68
  Response Record, 155, 156
  setting the stage for, 159–66, 189
  technique, 139, 145, 155, 156, 157, 167, 174, 189, 197, 198, 203, 206, 207, 209, 210, 211, 225, 231, 232, 276, 277, 279, 280, 281, 283, 285, 286, 288, 292, 341
  Technique, Learning the, an exercise, 146–51
  tension and, 142–57
  Tension Versus, an exercise, 144–45
Religion/Religious attitudes toward sex, 114, 249, 250, 258
Resentment, 99, 270
  and jealousy, 252–57

S

Scrotum, 73, 74, 121, 130
Self-consciousness, 23, 35, 113, 114, 131, 132, 133, 138, 140, 157, 269, 270, 273, 276, 279, 280, 282, 283, 285, 286, 289, 291, 293, 297, 322, 338
Self-discovery, 37–76, 77
Self-restraint, 110, 113, 114, 129, 131, 132, 133, 138, 197
Sensitivity:
  sexual, of men, 2, 5, 6, 7, 8, 11, 20, 21, 40, 41, 43, 52, 70, 75, 76, 105, 174, 195, 203, 241, 242
Sensual massage, 168, 175, 189, 201, 244, 245, 278, 279, 280, 281, 282, 283, 286, 287, 289, 290, 292, 302, 325, 326, 329
  Practicing, an exercise, 169–74
Sensuality, men's, 14, 20, 21, 43, 70–76
Separation (of spouses), 65, 250, 252, 293

Sex:
  a taboo subject in our culture, 133
  aggressive, as "best" sex, 30–31
  as achievement, 3, 20, 22, 72
  as bad, 130
  as conquest, 72
  as "dirty," 109, 114, 122, 130, 191, 205, 251
  as disgusting, 114, 205
  as shameful, 251
  as sinful, 109, 122, 130, 191, 193, 205, 248, 251
  as wrong, 114, 193, 248, 249, 268
  counseling, 193, 194, 290
  dislike of, 99–100
  drive, 2, 5, 21, 43, 84, 242
  fear of, 18, 110, 268, 299
  gentle, 31
  in the morning preferred, 101, 102
  intense, 31
  late at night preferred, 101
  liberated from reproduction, 18
  limited to late at night, 339
  loss of interest in, 12, 32, 33, 65, 69, 80, 118
  oral, 257, 340
  passionate, 31, 110, 308
  recreational, 61, 62, 63, 87
  reduced to a genital experience, 119
  roles, 2, 4, 41, 70, 71, 143
  therapists, 23, 29, 38, 70, 79, 84, 125, 233, 236, 264, 290, 307
  therapists, amateur, 302
  therapy, 32, 34, 65, 236, 239, 245, 262, 266
  therapy centers, 301
  therapy programs, 302
  violent, 30, 31
Sexual Activity Checklist, 93, 94–95, 96, 97
Sexual Activity Coding Sheet, 93, 94, 96, 97
Sexual communication, 78–92, 141, 175, 179, 280, 282, 343
  clear, 90
  inhibitions and, 92
  learning, 85–90
  open, 84
  overcoming fears of, 90
  negative, 78, 81
  nonverbal, 79, 90–92
  positive, 78, 81
  skills, 100, 105, 225, 279
  verbal, 79, 90, 91
Sexual desire, 40, 44, 52, 58, 59, 62, 63, 64, 69, 75, 110, 238, 245, 257, 258, 260, 268
  and erection problems, 240–42, 248
  erect penis a symbol of, 234
  loss of, 35, 139, 270
  relation of physical appearance to, 48, 49, 50
  versus moral values, 111
Sexual difficulties, 12, 32, 34, 195, 197, 199, 200, 201, 202, 203, 233, 252, 255, 261, 266, 293, 294, 298, 300, 338 (see also Sexual dysfunction; Sexual problems)
Sexual dysfunction, 1, 18, 35, 40, 42, 80, 193, 194, 196, 199, 204, 233, 236, 237, 239, 240, 243, 252, 255, 270, 273, 291, 307, 336 (see also Sexual difficulties; Sexual problems)
  and sexual scripts, 6–17
  cured in context of self-pleasure, 23
  implication of failed relationship in, 31–34
  in women, 14
  personal immaturity and, 32, 33
  Process, diagrammed, 271
  versus sexual fulfillment, 17–26
  vulnerability to, 17
Sexual encounters, 3, 5, 7, 16, 21, 35, 39, 43, 71, 72, 75, 80, 98, 99, 103, 104, 105, 108, 110, 113, 133, 141, 168, 174, 194, 199, 201, 202, 203, 232, 233, 234, 236, 245, 246, 247, 255, 257, 258, 261, 267, 272, 275, 276, 278, 284, 285, 289, 293, 295, 297, 299, 300, 301, 306, 308, 309, 311, 324, 334, 341

Sexual encounters (*cont.*)
  aggressive, 31
  bringing positive attitude to, 188
  communicating openly during, 82
  detecting nervous tension during, 158, 159
  difficulty relaxing during, 157
  erections and, 6, 32, 238–39, 269
  fantasy during, 123, 125
  fear of novelty in, 83
  foreplay, afterplay, and, 12
  frequency of specific activities during, 97
  genitally focused, 175, 176, 189
  male avoidance of, 10
  male responsibility during, 13, 14, 15, 22, 140
  minimizing discomfort during, 79
  mutual pleasure the motive for, 61
  preludes to, 5, 160, 162, 165–67, 189
  setting for, 100–101
Sexual expression:
  facilitating, 129–33
Sexual Fantasy Record, 126–28
Sexual fulfillment, 40, 63, 70, 76, 79, 84, 98, 100, 101, 106, 107, 108, 110, 129, 250, 265, 289, 334, 335
  and overall quality of relationships, 189
  lack of, 35
  patterns of intimacy and, 174–88
  sexual myths a barrier to, 240
  versus being functional, 17–26
Sexual history, 133–38, 253
  disclosing one's, 199–204
  Outline, 136–38
  sharing information about one's, 299
  Sharing Your, an exercise, 135–38
Sexual Interest, 75, 241
  Character and, an exercise, 52–59
  dimensions of, 43–70
  Physical Attributes and, an exercise, 44–52
  Relationships and, an exercise, 59–65
  schema, 310
  Specialness and, an exercise, 65–69
Sexuality:
  adult education courses in male, 37, 38
  assumptions about, 37
  changing one's attitudes about male, 196–97
  cultural constraints on, 108
  further development of, 107–38
  ideas concerning, 1
  lectures, workshops, etc., on, 108
  reassessing male and female, 1–36
  stereotypes about male, 41, 69
  traditional ideas about male, 44
  traditional views of, 21, 35
Sexual phobias, 191, 204–6, 232, 257, 258
Sexual preferences, 42, 43, 44, 45, 48, 49, 50, 52, 56, 69, 75, 76, 79, 80, 81, 89, 105, 179
  communicating one's, 91
  concerning the sexual situation, 101, 102, 105
  "modeling" of, 91
Sexual problems, 7, 12, 34, 191, 196, 202, 235, 237, 266, 293, 302
Sexual relationships, 2, 4, 12, 24, 25, 33, 34, 38, 42, 43, 66, 69, 71, 76, 93, 108, 109, 112, 119, 141, 157, 160, 161, 163, 165, 166, 174, 181, 194, 202, 204, 231, 232, 233, 234, 235, 245, 246, 247, 248, 256, 259, 262, 264, 266, 278, 282, 284, 289, 290, 291, 294, 298, 299, 300, 301, 302, 303, 304, 308, 315, 316, 335, 338, 340
  and Sexual Interest, an exercise, 59–65
  change and, 39, 40, 77, 78, 85, 111, 112, 141, 175
  dissatisfaction with, 17, 18
  dysfunction an implication of failed, 31–34

Sexual relationships (*cont.*)
  enhancing one's, 77–106, 107
  extramarital, 251
  ideals with respect to, 26
  intimacy in, 175, 176, 185, 187, 197
  kinds of, 59, 62
  nature of, 44
  potential of, 21
  priorities in, 162
  quality of, 70, 336
  relaxation and, 188, 189
  satisfaction with, 19
  schema, 62, 63
  sensual massage as part of, 173
  traditional pattern of, 13, 17
  unsatisfying, 23, 29
  variety of sexual activities in, 92
Sexual repertoires:
  balanced, 93, 98, 99, 100, 105
  broad, 93, 100, 105
  changing one's, 100
  expanding, 92–100, 175, 341
  narrow, 92
  reevaluating, 105
  sensual massage included in, 168
  unbalanced, 93
Sexual schemas:
  versus sexual scripts, 39–43
Sexual scripts:
  and sexual dysfunction, 6–17
  as "natural," 31
  breaking free of, 17, 19, 21, 39, 75, 265
  female, 4–6, 10, 15, 17, 21
  limitations of, 31, 35, 40, 72, 79
  lovemaking according to, 19, 79
  male, 2–4, 10, 12, 13, 14, 20, 25, 37, 44, 82, 101, 140, 158, 194, 297
  oppressive, 13
  restrictive, 80
  traditional, 71
  versus sexual schemas, 39–43
Sexual Self-Disclosure, an exercise, 199–204
Sexual Shyness, 42, 54, 131, 191–204, 247, 266, 293
  Understanding Your, an exercise, 192–99
Sexual Situation, 78, 100–105, 160, 241, 311
  Chart, 102, 103, 104
  Your Preferred, an exercise, 101–105
Sexual unfulfillment, 17, 18, 80, 93
Shame, 6, 10, 87, 109, 110, 113, 114, 115, 130, 131, 181, 193, 205, 233, 251, 307
Sharing:
  and Intimacy, an exercise, 185–88
  of feelings, 187, 188, 267
  of sexual fantasies, 135
  past sexual experiences, 134–35, 299
  pleasant experiences, 181
  responsibility for sexual satisfaction, 22, 23, 24, 25, 35, 39, 77, 80, 82, 84, 105, 141, 157, 164, 175, 186, 265
  responsibility for solving problems, 167
Single men:
  erection problems and, 297–304, 316
Singles' culture, 12
Specialness, 61
  and Sexual Interest, an exercise, 65–69
Spontaneity, 15
Stereotypes:
  about male sexuality, 41, 69
  of "beautiful" women, 44–45
Stimulation, 14, 41, 73, 88, 89, 91, 125, 236, 238, 273, 275, 280, 281, 283, 286, 309, 325, 333, 336, 337
  and Pause Record, 316–24, 327
  channels of, and sexual arousal, 310–14, 315, 338, 342, 344
  direct, 5, 14, 16, 21, 98, 99, 104, 123, 125, 314
  intense, 344
  manual, 118, 287, 326, 329
  of clitoris, 28, 30, 230
  oral, of male genitals, 84

Stimulation (*cont.*)
  photos as a source of, 208
  psychic, 3, 13, 14, 16, 21, 98, 99, 123, 125, 133, 314
  self-, 122, 281, 282, 315, 316, 317, 318, 319, 320, 321, 322, 324, 328, 340
  "shuttling" between sources of, 128
  sources of, 334
Strip poker, 292
Suppression, 110, 129, 142, 143
"Surrogates," 301

T

Taboos, 108, 109, 113, 114, 120, 133
Tension, 82, 190, 198, 201, 203, 205, 207, 209, 211, 212, 215, 216, 218, 219, 221, 222, 224, 276, 279, 280, 281, 285, 286, 288, 302, 341
  and relaxation, 142–57
  buildup of, 159
  chronic, 156, 167, 168
  detecting, 155–56
  detecting low levels of, 152
  extreme, 152
  overcoming sexual, 158–89
  reducing, 155
  -Relaxation Checklist, 152, 153
  release of, 159
  Versus Relaxation, an exercise, 144–45
Testicles, 288
Touching, 3, 41, 72, 79, 80, 91, 165, 173, 174, 191, 216, 218, 219, 220, 221, 222, 225, 226, 229, 257, 274, 282, 283, 285, 286, 288, 292, 318, 342, 343

Tubal ligation, 245
Turning down:
  sexual requests, 10, 89

U

Unhappiness, 1, 33, 40, 42

V

Vagina, 28, 244, 262, 283, 285, 286, 287, 289, 326, 329, 343
  capable of contraction and expansion, 230
  coloring of, 208
  congestion of, 118
  ejaculating outside, 133
  folds of, 208, 223
  inner lips of, 223
  lips of, 214
  lubrication of, 230, 328, 332
  opening of, 223
  outer lips of, 208, 214, 223, 229, 230
  shrinking of, 118
Vasectomy, 245
Venereal disease, 114
Vibrators, 29, 201, 274, 279, 280, 281, 282, 286, 287, 288, 340, 342
Violence, sexual, 30, 31
Virginity, 5, 83, 253
  male, 83
Virility:
  eagerness to prove, 195, 235
  questioning one's, 234
Vulnerability:
  of men, 41, 42